Set Point

I couldn't do it without you…thank you girls!

Set Point

Your Guide to Healthy Weight Maintenance

THOMAS MAZZONE MD

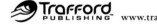 www.trafford.com

North America & international
toll-free: 1 888 232 4444 (USA & Canada)
phone: 250 383 6864 ♦ fax: 250 383 6804 ♦ email: info@trafford.com

The United Kingdom & Europe
phone: +44 (0)1865 722 113 ♦ local rate: 0845 230 9601
facsimile: +44 (0)1865 722 868 ♦ email: info.uk@trafford.com

10 9 8 7 6 5 4 3 2

Contents

There is of course only one way to take care of anything and that is to give it proper food and motions. And the motions that are akin to the divine in us are the thoughts and revolutions of the universe.

Plato in <u>*Timaeus*</u>

Introduction

Set Point is not a diet book. Instead it is a discussion about the reasons behind the obesity epidemic in North America. Why is it so difficult to maintain our weight, and can we do anything about it? I call it weight maintenance because weight loss is just the first step to a change in diet that results in a healthier life.

I realize that most of us would prefer to use some cookbook approach that guarantees weight loss. Wouldn't it be great to lose weight quickly and with minimal effort on our part? Maybe we should just eat the foods bought from certain weight loss programs—for a lot of money. Better yet why don't we all hire cooks and personal trainers who will be at our beckoned call, just like the media stars? Lest we forget—this is the real world. Fortunately there is a simple solution.

At any given time 60% of Americans express the desire to lose weight and 35% are actually dieting. According to the May 2004 National Institute of Nutrition report, 39% of Canadian women and 27% of men admitted to being on a diet. We obviously recognize that we have a problem. A few years ago two large circulation magazines, Time and National Geographic ran cover stories about obesity in America. Our expanded girths affect all aspects of our lives. For example, have you noticed that hotels now have bowed-out shower curtains to accommodate their larger customers? In 2000 the airlines spent $275 million more in fuel costs (as compared to 1990) to carry the additional weight of passengers. Do you honestly believe it will be possible to increase automobile fuel efficiency while making cars bigger so we fit in them comfortably? Since 2002, sales of "oversized" coffins[1] in Canada have increased four-fold.

An article in Toronto's <u>Globe and Mail</u> revealed that a 2004 plane crash into the icy waters of Lake Erie was caused by the weight of the eight passengers on board. "The aircraft's occupants, including their carry-on baggage, each weighed an average of about 240 pounds (108 kilograms)—30% more than the regulations allowed."[2] A recently released Duke University study found that overweight workers lost 13 times more work days, resulting in seven times higher medical claims, than their fit co-workers.[3]

We consume diet books by the dozens, all of which promise deliverance from this epidemic. In 2001 the <u>New York Times</u> proclaimed that books about food had replaced books about sex on its best-seller list. I will bet that this is not the first book about weight loss that you have read. Look at your own bookshelf. Dr. Atkins or Dr. Phil? Low carb or low fat? The Zone or the Maker? Counting points or counting calories? We have heard of and perhaps even tried them all, but have these weight loss plans had any impact? Let's look at the statistics.

In the latest, large scale U.S. government survey 97 million adults were overweight (67% of men, 62% of women), with 44

---

[1] Coffins that are 68-72 cm (26.5 to 29 inches) wide. A standard unit is 61 cm (24 inches).

[2] <u>The Globe and Mail</u>, Saturday, December 10, 2005, Page 1.

[3] Ostbye, T., et al: "Obesity and Worker's Compensation". <u>Archives of Int. Med</u>, April 2007,167: 766-773. 183 days lost vs. 14 per full-time equivalents and $51,178 vs. $7503 per 100 FTE!

million being classified obese.[4] Canadian statistics aren't much better: in 2004 59% were overweight with 23% being obese. Obesity is defined as weighing more than 30% over an ideal weight. Think about wearing a backpack containing at least one-third of your recommended weight. No wonder you feel weighed down—to say nothing about the other deleterious effects on health and well-being. Obesity and its complications—diabetes and heart disease—add more than $100 billion (over 9% of the total) to our yearly health care costs.[5] All medical problems are worsened, for example obese patients who suffer major trauma have a seven times greater chance of dying while in the hospital. A study from Denmark found that obese couples took three times longer to get pregnant.[6]

Originally the Center for Disease Control had estimated that 400,000 Americans died annually from obesity and its complications, more than those killed by alcohol (85,000), car accidents (43,000) and guns (29,000) combined. The CDC then decreased its estimate so that obesity now only kills 112,000 Americans annually, still making it the 7th leading cause of preventable death.[7] According to representatives from the National Center for Health Statistics this change was the result of a more accurate or revised interpretation of statistical data—not new data (hmmm).

No matter how you interpret the statistics the numbers are still unacceptable. For some reason though, we don't truly express

---

[4] Third National Health and Nutrition Examination Survey (NHANES III), 1991.

[5] In 1986 these numbers were $39.3 billion or 5% of the yearly total.

[6] Ramlau-Hansen, C., et al. Human Reproduction, March 7, 2007.

[7] "Excess Deaths Associated With Underweight, Overweight and Obesity," Katherine Flegal, et. al., JAMA 2005; 293: p. 1861.

our outrage. There has been no drive to ban snack food or fast food ads on TV like there was for tobacco. There is no anti-obesity lobby in Washington like the anti-gun lobby. The police don't ticket people sitting in front of a huge plate of food like they do when they drive without a seat belt. Where are the Mothers Against Obese Kids (MAOK) demonstrating to increase awareness about the toll food takes on their children like the Mothers Against Drunk Drivers (MADD)?

Obesity increases the risk of cardiovascular disease (CVD) by increasing cholesterol, increasing circulating fat and thickening the blood. One half of obese adults have high blood pressure, which is a major risk factor for CVD[8]. 80% of the deaths from diabetes are the result of CVD. The rate of diabetes in the US has gone up 67% (from 2.8% to 4.2%) in the last 20 years, and it has been estimated that undiagnosed diabetes exists in another 5.2 million Americans.

The direct medical costs related to diabetes have risen from $44 billion in 1997 to $92 billion in 2002. While all these statistics are alarming enough, check out what's happening to our children.

Most experts believe that this next generation will be the first generation of Americans whose life expectancy is shorter than their parents. <u>What are you leaving your children</u>? Talk about a death tax! Consider that Type 2 diabetes, once virtually unknown in this age group, has doubled in the children of certain population groups. If diabetes is diagnosed before the age of 15, your child will lose 17 to 27 years from her life. About 40% of kids ages 5 to 8 carry at least one risk factor for CVD. The World Heart Federation warned that obese children have a three to five time's greater risk than normal weight children of suffering heart attack or stroke before age 65. In the US, 13.7% of children under the age of eleven and 11.5%

---

[8] 61.8 million Americans have CVD, causing 1 of every 2.5 deaths in US, and costing $351.8 billion annually.

of adolescents are obese. These percentages have doubled in the last 20 years. How did it come to this?

According to government statistics, 40 years ago the average man in the US weighed 166 pounds. Today he has ballooned to 191 pounds, an increase of 25 pounds (+15%). Women have gained even more, from 140 to 164 pounds, a jump of 24 pounds (+17%). In the last 25 years the Canadian man has gone from 167 to 182 pounds (+9%) and woman from 138 to 153 (+11%). The reason is obvious. The Center of Disease Control has reported that from 1971 to 2000, the average woman increased her daily calories by 22% (from 1,542 to 1,877 or by 335 calories). The average man increased his intake by 7% (from 2,450 to 2,618 calories or 168 calories). Compare these values to those recommended by the government: 1,600 calories for women and 2,200 calories for men. When the data was further analyzed, besides the increase in calories, researchers found that empty calories accounted for almost one-third of the total.[9]

At what age does this problem begin? Another study[10] found that the average child between 1 and 2 years old consumed 1,220 calories daily. This is 28% above the government recommendation of 950 calories. Remarkably, even infants between 7 and 11 months consumed 20% more calories daily than recommended! Most nutritionists (and psychologists) agree that eating habits are established by age 3.

As if all those extra calories weren't enough, we have also gotten much less active. I prefer not to use the term—exercise too little—because that makes it seem as if we have to run,

[9] "Foods contributing to energy intake in the US," Gladys Block, Journal of Food Composition and Analysis, June 2004, p. 439: 12.3% from sweets and desserts, 7.1% from soft drinks, 5% from salty snacks and sweet drinks, and 4.4% from alcohol.

[10] The Feeding Infants and Toddlers Study (FITS)

swim or bicycle more. The fact is that we have become too sedentary. In 1924, 87% of women did more than four hours of housework daily, in 1977 that number dropped to 43% and in 1999 only 14% of women continued to work so slavishly at home. For men the decrease in old economy jobs such as mining, factory and even farm work has resulted in similar decreases in activity. 40 years ago Americans spent 20% of their income on food, today that percentage has shrunk to less than 10%. While these changes are an admirable consequence of our increasing affluence, when you can afford to eat more calories and you burn up less, the results are predictable.

Our suburban sprawl with its increased reliance on the automobile has also made us less active. A study from the National Center for Smart Growth at the University of Maryland found that those who lived in the least populated, most sprawling counties weighed 6 pounds more than those who lived in Manhattan. The reason for the difference was that city dwellers are forced to walk more. Only 17% of our school children walk to school. By the age of 17 the average child has spent more time sitting in front of the TV than attending school. <u>Less than 25% of American kids get 30 minutes of any type of physical exercise daily</u>. One out of four school children does not attend gym class.[11] Researchers from the University of Chicago have concluded that if kindergartners engaged in 5 hours of physical activity per week (the amount recommended by the US government), there would be a decrease in obesity of 43%.

In conclusion, the reason that we are overweight and continue to add to the problem is that <u>we eat too much and do not move around enough</u>. It is that simple! Throw away all those other excuses: "It's my genes...I don't have time to cook...my

---

[11] A decrease of 10% in only 10 years. What a sad comment if the reason behind this decrease is, as the experts believe, the fear of liability on the part of the school boards.

metabolism is different...I have to cook for my whole family, and they don't eat vegetables...it's the holidays." Eat less and exercise more! Those are the secrets to weight maintenance. How do you begin?

The first chapter of <u>Set Point</u> will discuss how we look at food. Attitude is all! <u>The relationship between food and culture is the most important, yet overlooked, determinant of weight loss and gain</u>. The next chapter will present the 10 Commandments of weight maintenance. The following chapters will explain the Commandments, some of which will be detailed separately while others will be discussed together. It will become obvious that they are actually all interrelated. The chapter on Set Point will offer an explanation about weight loss and maintenance. The reasons are pretty straight forward and they center on metabolism, evolution and survival. Afterwards I will detail an easy, inexpensive diet plan that changes your Set Point.

1

Food and Culture

As the introduction stated, the simplest explanation for the rise in obesity is that we eat too much, and exercise too little. Address those two points and you solve the problem. However, I understand it's not that easy. There are many other things that come into play. It is obvious that obesity runs in families, i.e. overweight parents have overweight kids. In fact it has been found that children born to obese mothers are almost three times more likely to be overweight by the age of 4 and twice as likely by the age of 2.[1] This fact condemns the child to a life of weight problems. The average 10 year old weighs 11 pounds more than he did in 1960. Unfortunately, statistics demonstrate that if childhood obesity continues into adolescence, 80% will remain obese as adults. It is not known how much of this "inheritance" is related to genetics, and how much is related to poor eating habits.

---

[1] 24% of children were obese if mother was obese during first three months of pregnancy vs. 9% if mother was of normal weight. Even worse, as reported in the December 5, 2005 Pediatrics, if a woman was overweight before she became pregnant her child was three times more likely to be overweight by age 7 compared to children from normal weight mothers.

The FITS study found that kids' food preferences are pretty much established by the age of 3. You may be shocked by what the researchers discovered:

- Almost one-third of children under age 2 ate no vegetables, and of those who did, the most common vegetable cited over the age of 15 months were French fries.
- 9% kids 9-11 months ate French fries daily, 20% kids 19 months to 2 years ate French fries daily.
- 7% kids 9-11 months and 25% over 15 months ate hot dogs, sausage or bacon daily.
- More than 60% of the younger group and 75% of the older group had dessert or candy daily.
- 30-40% of children over 15 months had a sugary fruit drink daily and almost 10% drank soda pop.

How can anyone consider deep fried, trans-fat and starch laden French fries a healthy vegetable? Yet the statistics show parents serving them as such. We have been inundated by commercials selling fruit juice and sugary fruit drinks as good things to serve your kids, yet we ignore the research that says pre-schoolers who drank more than 12 ounces of juice (any juice) per day are at increased risk of being short and obese. Bottled and canned juices are pasteurized (destroying nutrients and enzymes), acidic (affecting muscle functioning) and reduce the child's appetite for whole foods.

Consider the following about the eating patterns of children:

- The top sources of calories in America are milk, soda pop, white bread, sugar, ground beef, white flour and processed cheese.
- The most popular items in school cafeterias are fast foods, pizza, potato chips and baked and frozen desserts.

- The National School Lunch Program has a mandate to provide a market for surplus foodstuffs—particularly beef and dairy products.
- Many teachers use candy or pizza parties to reward their classes.
- World-wide the consumption of soft drinks has been proven to increase calorie consumption, increase body weight, decrease other necessary nutrients and increase the risk of diabetes.
- The risk of obesity increases 1.6 times for each soda pop consumed.
- There has been a 500% increase in high sugar beverages in the last 50 years.
- From 1985 to 1997 school districts increased their purchase of soda pop 1100%
- Hundreds of school districts have signed contracts with soft drink companies for the exclusive right to sell their soft drinks.
- Soft drinks now account for over 10% of the average adolescent's calories.
- There are over 3 million soft drink vending machines in the U.S.

Although always wary of governmental micro-managing, we seem to ignore the fact that our tastes are fashioned by the food industry and by the media:

- The average 17 year old has spent more time watching TV than attending school—it's not even close![2]
- The more TV they watch, the more food our kids consume.
- The risk of obesity rises 6% for every hour a child watches TV.
- The average child watches 40,000 commercials yearly, working out to 10 food commercials each hour.

---

[2] 18,000 hours watching TV vs. 12,000 hours in class.

- On Saturday morning TV, 71% of commercials are for food, with over 90% of those hawking fast foods, sugary cereals, cookies, chips, candy, sugary fruit drinks or soda.

We're afraid to let our children walk to the school bus yet who's concerned when the food industry spends almost $3 billion yearly to sell them products, half of which are for fat and calorie laden foods? Every parent should imitate the people in the movie "Network", throw open your windows and shout: "I'm mad as hell and I'm not going to take it anymore!"

Welcome changes

The word is getting out:

- Addressing growing concern over the rise of obesity in children in France, Parliament ignored lobbying by the food industry and voted to ban all vending machines that sell sweets and soft drinks in French schools.
- In October, 2004, the government of Ontario, Canada banned the sale of junk-food from elementary-school vending machines.
- In September, 2005 Governor Arnold Schwarzenegger terminated the use of sugary sodas in California schools.
- English celebrity chef Jamie Oliver has led a campaign to replace the fatty, salty, greasy, sugary food in Britain's schools with freshly cooked, nutritious meals.
- On May 3, 2006 the beverage industry announced voluntary restrictions on selling sugary drinks to school children. Sodas, diet sodas, sports drinks, juice drinks, apple and grape juice would no longer be sold in elementary schools.

- In June 2007 Kellogg Co. said that all of its products will be reformulated to meet new health standards[3] or they won't be advertised to children.

More needs to be done. It is well-known that socio-economic status also has a marked influence on obesity. In our distant past, fatness denoted success and affluence. It fostered survival especially through hard times. In the Bible it was written: "Those that be planted in the house of the Lord...shall be fat and flourishing."[4] Today, how things have changed.

Obesity is commonly associated with poverty and lower socio-economic status. One in four adults below the poverty level is obese versus one in six in households earning over $67,000. While 13.7% of all children are obese, those numbers increase to 16% in black, non-Hispanic and 17% in Mexican-Americans. A new study calls obesity "the new malnutrition" with 42% homeless children in Baltimore, Maryland either overweight or at risk for being overweight and 77% of their care-caregivers obese or overweight.[5]   It's not hard to figure out why this is true. Studies have shown that the poor watch more TV. For many families, television is the baby-sitter, or at least the entertainer. Also cheaper foods tend to be higher in fat and carbohydrates. For example, Mexican-Americans eat a diet laced with corn. Tortillas are the number two grain product consumed in America, after bread. In conclusion, the poor tend to consume more calories, saturated fat, soft drinks, refried grains and meat, and are less active.

---

[3] Maximum 200 calories per serving, no trans fat, 2 g saturated fat, 12 g sugar, 230 mg salt.

[4] Psalm 92: 13, 14.

[5] Medscape General Medicine (3/07/2007).

Farm policy

The plot thickens: consider U.S. farm policy. In 1930 American farmers produced 1.8 trillion bushels of corn and this number has doubled every 30 years since. Today they produce 10 trillion bushels. This increased production has been both the farmer's friend and worst enemy. The marketplace is flooded with grain, and the price therefore is correspondingly low, forcing the farmer to grow more, which drives the price down even lower. The US government props up the farmers with $19 billion in subsidies per year. Everyone wants a part of this largess. Agribusiness sees the profit potential and develops genetically altered seeds that are more disease resistant and will produce more per acre.[6] So what do we do with the surplus corn? Turn it into easier to store and use, value-added commodities: high-fructose corn syrup (the ingredient of choice in soda, sweetened juices, sports drinks, candy, ketchup, and most processed foods), and feed for our livestock (beef, pork and chicken).

The next time you happen to be waiting at a railroad crossing take a look at what is written on many of the black tanker cars that make up many trains—high fructose corn syrup. In my boredom once I counted 62 tanker cars of corn syrup in one train! I have to quote from an article by Michael Pollan in the New York Times Magazine:

> Cheap corn, the dubious legacy of Earl Butz[7], is truly the building block of the "fast-food nation."

---

[6] One of the big international trade policy issues today is the refusal on the part of many countries to allow the importation of genetically altered grains. I do not believe that this choice is being made solely on protectionism. No one really knows what altering the genetic code of food products (humans?) will do to future generations.

[7] President Nixon's Secretary of Agriculture who encouraged farmers to overproduce corn inaugurating a new Federal subsidy program. This drove down the price of corn and thereby controlled commodity prices which

Cheap corn, transformed into high-fructose corn syrup, is what allowed Coca-Cola to move from the svelte 8-ounce bottle of soda ubiquitous in the 70's to the chubby 20-ounce bottle of today. Cheap corn, transformed into cheap beef, is what allowed McDonald's to supersize its burgers and still sell many of them for no more than a dollar. Cheap corn gave us a whole raft of highly processed foods, including the world-beating chicken nugget, which, if you study its ingredients, you discover is really a most ingenious transubstantiation of corn, from the corn-fed chicken it contains to the bulking and binding agents that hold it together.

To prevent cheap corn from lowering the price of food too much, the food industry decided to increase the average portion size. It's not just a coincidence that we eat so many more calories than before. Interestingly, research has shown that humans will eat what is set down in front of them, regardless of portion size, i.e. bigger portions, eat more calories.[8]

Recently more people have become aware of the danger of corn and similar grain products through the low-carb craze. Corn and corn products have some of the highest glycemic (GI) index foods. The South Beach Diet tries to avoid high GI foods. Yet the subtle and not so subtle addition of corn to processed food is difficult to avoid. The only alternative is to wean yourself and your family off processed foods. Can you imagine if the public brought pressure onto the government and the food industry and demanded healthier foods? What would agribusiness do with all the surplus corn?

---

enabled Nixon to sell grain to the Soviets in 1972 without driving up the price of food for the American consumer.

[8] Probably true with all animals—just watch how your dog will eat non-stop.

Obviously the government would never allow the market to collapse. Remember it already props up the industry with over $19 billion in subsidies. In the late 1970's, during the last "oil crisis", there was a movement to add ethanol (distilled from corn) to gasoline to make gasohol[9]. Because it costs more to produce, gasohol was not considered profitable until oil prices rose above $25-30 per barrel[10]. In 2002, 21 billion gallons of gasohol were produced. It has been estimated that gasohol displaces about 5% of the total gasoline used in the U.S. What if there was a mandate to displace 15-20% of the present gas supply? It would be a public-relations home-run if the Federal government became less dependent on foreign oil and encouraged (not subsidized) weight loss at the same time.

One last word about corn: in the last 20 years there has been a change in the strains of corn preferentially grown in the US. I ate a few ears of sweet corn recently and was amazed at the sweetness—it bordered on being sickening. Researching the trends I discovered that the sugar content has risen four-fold.[11] More sugar means increased shelf-life, more high-fructose corn syrup and ethanol production and ultimately, the manipulation of public taste.

You may ask yourself what this diversion into government policy has to do with losing weight. It is difficult, if not impossible to control your diet and the diets of your children without realizing that many of the foods that are bad for you are the direct result of present government policies. It seems a little disingenuous on the part of State and National legislators to sponsor "cheese-burger bills" (strongly supported by State restaurant associations) that prohibit people from suing food

---

[9] Gasohol is gasoline with 10% ethanol added to it.

[10] In February 2008 the price hit $102 per barrel.

[11] Sc2 strains have 22-40% sugar versus the old content of 5-11%.

manufacturers, sellers, and advertisers for claims arising from their weight gain, obesity and/or health related problems.

Don't get me wrong, I believe that the individual is ultimately responsible for her diet and consequent health decisions. However, the government makes policies that foster over-consumption, protects the businesses that benefit from that over-consumption, and then refuses to admit that there is a concerted effort driving over-consumption! To change dietary patterns requires an awareness of the reasons why our food is so cheap, readily available and so harmful to our health. "I'm mad as hell and I'm not going to take it anymore."

Fast-food nation

Present statistics show that weight gain is common in the entire "industrialized" world, but there is no denying that North America has one of the biggest problems. Is there something in our culture that contributes to our weight gain? What are other countries doing to address obesity? Stating the obvious, we exercise less than they do and we eat more. In a recent article in the Herald Tribune the author wrote:

> Europeans like to walk even when they have no place to go. An entire European family could make canapés from the staggering high pile of cold cuts in just one New York deli sandwich. Italians return from abroad stunned by cherished U.S. dining habits like all-you-can eat restaurants and doggy bags for all you can't eat.

I remember years ago eating in a famous steak house chain that had a salad bar. I grew up believing that salad was lettuce, tomato and sometimes other vegetables that were added to vary the mix. As I stood over the troughs of food I was amazed that various pastas, pizza, relishes and cheeses were available for unlimited consumption. It didn't take me long to notice the size of my fellow diners, or should I say grazers.

Most Europeans go out to dine, Americans increasingly just feed! In Italy, the "slow-food" movement began as a reaction against the invasion of fast-food into the country. One of the complaints against American fast-food chains in France is their seductive influence on their children. Happy clowns—happy meals—do you want a movie toy with your meal and excess calories?

There are over 170,000 fast-food restaurants in the U.S. and access to their high fat, high caloric foods seems to be on every street corner. The percentage of calories that our kids eat at home has declined from 82% in the late 70's to 68% in 1994, and the calories contributed by fast-food have risen from 2 to 15%. On days when kids eat fast food, they consume 187 more calories than on other days. <u>American kids eat fast-food one out of three days</u>. This year over 50% of Americans will eat at McDonalds at least once.

In his surprise hit "Super Size Me", filmmaker Morgan Spurlock ate three meals per day at McDonald's. Over one month's filming he gained 25 pounds and his cholesterol rose from 168 to 230. In an interview in the NY Times Spurlock said, "I was completely depressed, tired and lethargic, and I'd get these incredible headaches that would go away once I started eating the fast food again. My cholesterol skyrocketed, my blood pressure went up…and my liver was basically filling with fat…my liver was pâté."[12]

In some fascinating research coming out of the University at Buffalo,[13] Dr. Paresh Dondana reports that 3 hours after a high fat, 900 calorie fast-food breakfast deadly free radicals and inflammatory components percolate through the blood stream.

---

[12] Stunned by the criticism, to its credit, McDonald's moved quickly to update its menu with healthier choice options.

[13] News item, WGRZ TV, Buffalo, New York June 2006.

These substances have been implicated in the development of atherosclerosis (hardening of the arteries). The recommended use of vitamin C (versus free radicals) and aspirin (versus inflammation), are a testament to this knowledge. While there is a 200% increase in these toxic substances following a high fat meal, a meal of fruit and fiber (providing the same 900 calories) shows no increase at all.

According to a report by the European Food Safety Authority, Europeans eat less of the dangerous, cholesterol-raising fats than Americans do, and the amount is decreasing. The French consider a 12% obesity rate (compared to over 30% in the U.S.) a national health care emergency and they are actively taking steps to address the problem.[14] When the eating habits in France were analyzed it was noted that butter, soft cheeses and bread were daily staples. However, the French and Italians never eat a big breakfast, preferring instead a baguette with butter (not margarine), croissant or sweet roll and coffee. Often lunch is the largest meal of the day, with dinner being late and a little lighter. Importantly, most of the menu items begin with whole foods. The concept of low fat, chemically altered and enhanced or artificially sweetened foods is a North American invention.

X-food

We seem to have forgotten the importance of taste and proportion. Instead we have replaced them with extreme foods and eating. Note the increase of eating contests. First it was hot-dogs, then it was chicken wings and ham hocks, now its chili peppers.

---

[14] Banning soft drink vending machines was part of this initiative. The legislature is also debating whether to add a warning label on foods: **"Eating this product in large quantities can make you obese."**

Personally I don't think it's very appetizing or entertaining to watch people making pigs out of themselves. Hardee's sells a 1,420 calorie "Monster Thickburger". After Burger King introduced the 730 calorie, 47 grams of fat "Enormous Omelet Sandwich", its breakfast sales increased 20%. Seeing the effect on its bottom line, BK added a "Quad Stacker" which is a four-layered cheeseburger containing over 1000 calories and 68 grams of fat.[15] Even salads have become X-foods, for example the "Santa Fe Salad" at Arby's has 845 calories and 60 grams of fat.

I have often heard people complain that when they order pizza in Italy they are disappointed to find it thin and sparsely topped, especially with cheese. It's all about quality ingredients in the proper proportion—not putting an entire stick of pepperoni on top and extra cheese in the crust.

Dining not feeding

I recently ate a meal in France with some friends. Between courses they placed down their utensils and talked, so the meal lasted over two hours. During these breaks, my body worked its magic sending back cues that it was satisfied. Compare this to stopping at the drive-thru of a fast food restaurant, eating a large burger and fries and washing it down with a huge cola on the way to a meeting—supersize me! We just stuff ourselves without ever listening to what our bodies are telling us.

The debate about the eating habits of Americans keeps heating up. We analyze the minutia of our diets in search of the offending agents:

> Perhaps because we take a more "scientific" (i.e. reductionist) approach to food Americans

---

[15] Jeff Novick, director of nutrition for the Pritikin Longevity Center states: "This burger might better be called the quadruple-bypass special." Quoted in The Globe and Mail, November 4, 2006, page F7.

automatically assume there must be some chemical component that explains the difference between the French and American experiences: it's something in the red wine, perhaps, or the olive oil that's making them healthier. But <u>how we eat, and even how we feel about eating, may in the end be just as important as *what* we eat</u>.

The French eat all sorts of "unhealthy" foods, but they do it according to a strict and stable set of rules: they eat small portions and don't go back for seconds; they don't snack; they seldom eat alone, and communal meals are long, leisurely affairs<u>. A well-developed culture of eating, such as you find in France or Italy, mediates the eater's relationship to food, moderating consumption even as it prolongs and deepens the pleasure of eating.</u>[16]

According to the American Dietetic Association two out of three American workers spend their lunch hour at their desk. Among those who regularly ate lunch at their desks, 37% also ate breakfast and 61% have afternoon snacks in their office or cubicle. Slave to your work? A spokeswoman for the ADA was quoted: "If your mind is distracted, you don't get the full benefit of the meal. Your brain has to be satisfied." Satisfied? Most of us gulp down food without even knowing what we're eating. It's not much better for our kids. Considering the time it takes to get to the cafeteria, go through the food line and sit down, the average child eats lunch in 15 minutes! In Europe the lunch hour really does last 60 minutes.

One of the best (worst?) examples of fast-food consumption and eating while distracted is found in any large airport. Just sit and observe your fellow overweight travelers. Their pace is frenetic and the travel stress and fatigue is written on their

---

[16] Michael Pollan, <u>New York Times Magazine</u>, October 17, 2004.

faces. What do they do? Gobble down sugary buns, high-calorie coffee concoctions and pizza or nachos out of little plastic boxes. Recently I sat in an airport restaurant and watched a well-dressed elderly couple order a plate of gigantic onion rings and cheese-dripping quesadillas. After eating half the meal they stopped and looked aghast at what they had done. We truly are multi-tasking as we eat out of a bag while staring at the blaring airport TV, paging through our itineraries, talking on cell phones or typing on our laptops—sometimes all at once.

I can hear the collective groan now: "There isn't enough time!" I have already said that the solution is easy, but it would take a collective change of consciousness. Isn't your health important to you? Our health care costs are skyrocketing,[17] and in a poll conducted by the Harvard School of Public Health, 79% surveyed felt that obesity was a major health issue. Throwing money at the problem, taking expensive drugs or going through dangerous medical procedures doesn't seem to be the common sense approach. Some large companies like Sprint and Union Pacific are taking more aggressive measures to get their employees to lose weight, and adopt a healthier lifestyle. Analyzing injury claims and illness records, Union Pacific estimates that if the percentage of its overweight employees were reduced by just one point it would save $1.7 million; by 5%, save $8.5 million; and by 10%, save $16.9 million.

To solve the problem of eating too much requires a conscious effort to know what you are eating, and taking enough time to let the body do its work. According to the Committee for Health Education, 75% of the French eat dinner together as a family and many French schoolchildren still go home for lunch. In America the family meal is disappearing, on average only one family in three sits down and eats dinner together. Talk about

---

[17] In the U.S. health care consumes 16% GNP, double the average in other industrialized countries. It is expected to reach 20% GNP.

family values. <u>A University of Michigan study found that the family meal was the single strongest predictor of better achievement scores and fewer behavior problems in children</u>. Mealtime was more important than time spent in school, in church, playing sports or performing artistic activities. Children who eat with their parents consume more fruits and vegetables, less fried and fast food, and snack less often between meals.

Alice Waters, founder of Chez Panisse in Berkeley and the chef who redefined California cuisine stated in an interview with the <u>New York Times Magazine</u>:

> "We're losing the values we learned from our parents when we sat around our family table, when we lived closer to the land and communicated. The way children are eating now is teaching them about disposability, about sameness, about fast, cheap and easy. They learn that work is to be avoided, that preparation is drudgery."[18]

Walk about

I followed a school bus the other day down some long suburban street. It stopped at every other house dropping off kids as their mothers waved expectantly from their open front doors. It took 20 minutes to travel 2 miles! I am not going to relate the 10 miles each way to school—in the snow—uphill— story. But I do remember that I had to walk a mile or so to get to one of the designated bus-stops where other kids who walked a mile or so waited with me. Today, only 17% of our kids walk to school, and most of them can't seem to walk further than their driveway. I realize that changes have taken place in our society. The streets are busier and parents worry about the speeding traffic, to say nothing of the threat of abduction on the way to school or waiting for a bus. <u>Has it</u>

---

[18] March 7, 2004.

gotten so bad on our streets that our kids can't walk more than a few feet? Not exactly an endorsement of a safe citizenry! What exactly is homeland security?   Maybe the overweight parents could also get some exercise with their sedentary children. Oh yea, I remember—not enough time! All I can ask is what is important to you?

I watched the local news recently during which numerous mothers were interviewed in their SUVs about driving their kids around. The consensus was that they enjoyed the activity: not only could they keep their children safe, but they could spend quality time with them. "What else would I do with my time?" offered one mom. How about walking around the block or even eating together?

Another observation that I've had in my travels is the activity level of the local people. Americans have to schedule or find time to exercise. As I mentioned in the introduction I prefer not to use the term exercise because of the connotation.[19] In other countries people walk everywhere.   Even though public transportation is used—the people walk. Try riding the Metro in Paris all day: up and down stairs, transferring to other trains through long passageways and walking to the next Metro station. Once again that is why New Yorkers are thinner than their countrymen living in the suburban sprawl. In Italy there is a lovely tradition called the "passeggiata" (promenade) in which the streets of every city and town become filled with the locals out for an evening stroll. This same tradition exists in many other countries.   Americans seem to have an aversion to walking, or perhaps our way of living has made walking too difficult.

In most foreign cities you see people walking around carrying shopping bags. They walk to work, pass the farmer's market on the way home, and pick up something for dinner. When I mention this to people I usually try to show them the

---

[19] That it's something that must be worked into the daily schedule.

differences in our way of life by starting off: "They shop for food every day!" This gets a rise out of most North Americans who envision sitting in their minivan, waiting in traffic, fighting through the crowded supermarket with a huge cart overloaded with staples, hauling all the bags in and out of their vehicle, and doing it every day! Contrary to this frenetic activity, shopping for many of the city dwellers is the routine selection of what looks good that day.

While I am not advocating everyone give up their way of life, to change your diet require changes in attitudes. Fundamental attitudes at that! It's time to realize. It's time to recognize. It's time to mobilize:

- Realize that only you can change your dietary patterning.
- Recognize what choices you make.
- Mobilize to change.

Open the front door and walk—don't run—to the corner and back. It's a start.

2

Ten Commandments

1. All diets work. All diets are meant to fail.

2. What's good for your health is good for your diet.

3. To be successful a diet needs to be balanced and offer variety.

4. The best diet would be simple: low cost, readily available foods that are easy to prepare.

5. Don't try to fake out your body! Eat real food.

6. Knowledge is power. Know what you eat.

7. You didn't gain the weight overnight, so don't expect to lose it overnight.

8. Don't drink your calories.

9. Walk more.

10. To change your set point you must change your mindset! Be honest with yourself.

3

The Diet Dilemma

Let's begin with the First Commandment: **All diets will work.
All diets are meant to fail.** Talk to anyone you know and they
will tell you about some miracle diet that they're trying, or about
the difficulty they are having with losing weight on the diet that
everyone else succeeds. What's going on? Remember the
cabbage soup diet, the lettuce diet, the hot dog diet? How
about the raw foods diet? They have all been touted as the
next best thing.

How we look at specific foods continues to evolve. To the
Romans, barbarians were people who didn't eat bread; to the
Chinese they didn't eat rice. In 1825 the French lawyer, Jean
Anthelme Brillat-Savarin, wrote about the benefits of eating a
diet low in carbohydrates in the book The Physiology of Taste.
His message fell in and out of favor for 150 years, until Dr.
Robert Atkins reestablished interest in limiting carbohydrate
intake in his book Dr. Atkin's Diet Revolution. It has recently
been estimated that 26 million Americans are on a low-carb
diet.   The business of low-carb foods, diet books, and
supplements will generate $30 billion dollars this year. Isn't it
interesting that since the Atkins diet was proposed in 1972 we

haven't gotten any thinner? Perhaps the low-carb craze is just another fad.[1]

In a cover article in the <u>New York Times Magazine</u>, Dr. David Katz, nutrition spokesman for the American College of Preventative Medicine asked: "What if it's all been a big fat lie?" He argued that any diet that doesn't address the simple problem of eating more calories than we're burning up, will ultimately fail. The bottom line: calories do matter! Another concern about Atkins is that no distinction is made between good fats and bad. Most health care practitioners agree that eating 15 pieces of bacon and processed cheese is not good for your health.   We all realize this fact. After her husband's heart surgery, Sen. Hillary Clinton was quoted on Good Morning America[2] as questioning the former President about adopting a low carb diet: "I didn't think it was healthy...I'd say, 'You really think you should have a cheeseburger every day for lunch?'" She had begun to worry about his health when he became fatigued on walks.

Concerns over the safety of the Atkins diet spawned the <u>South Beach Diet</u> (by the way—it was the diet President Clinton was following) which distinguishes between good and bad carbohydrates (not just low-carb).   It advises avoiding high glycemic index foods.[3] The problem, as noted by Dr. Katz, is that some of the choices made using this criterion don't make a whole lot of sense, for example carrots have a higher glycemic index than ice cream.

The Weight and Eating Disorders Program at the University of Pennsylvania, School of Medicine conducted the first head-to-head trial of the four most popular diet plans: Atkins, Dr.

---

[1] How fickle we are! On August 1, 2005 Atkins Nutritionals declared bankruptcy due to declining sales of its packaged food line.

[2] ABC News, Friday October 29, 2004.

[3] Those that raise blood sugar too quickly, especially important in diabetics

Ornish's <u>Eat More, Weigh Less</u>, Weight Watchers and <u>The Zone</u>. All those who stayed on their diet for one year had comparable weight loss (5% or 10 pounds for someone weighing 200 pounds). If they went on a diet, but did not stay on it for the entire year, their weight loss averaged 3% (6 pounds for a 200 pound person). Sounds pretty meager when compared to the guarantees given in the ads you will find in any magazine of 10 pounds in two weeks! The more extreme diets, Atkins (very low carb) and Ornish (very low fat) lost about half their participants over the year while the Zone and Weight Watchers lost about a third. The drop-out rate is even worse in Great Britain where 13% of people responded that they had tried the Atkins diet, but only 3% stayed on it. One benefit of <u>all</u> the diets was a significant (average 10%) drop in the risk of heart attack, mainly related to an improvement in blood lipids.[4]

Another study just released in the <u>Journal of the American Medical Association</u> found that the Atkins diet <u>was</u> the most successful but as the author Dr. Christopher Gardner was quoted: "Atkins did double the weight loss (compared to the other diets), but how excited can you get about 10 pounds of weight loss over the course of a year? I'm worried this study is going to get abused. Stories are going to say, 'Here's the solution to the obesity epidemic. Atkins has been vindicated.' That is really not what we found."[5]

If these are the most popular diets, and they generate only modest success, how can anyone stay motivated, lose weight, and keep it off? That is the diet dilemma: while most diets will work, they eventually will fail. <u>The simplest explanation is that if you do not change the habits that got you fat in the first place, nothing will fundamentally change</u>.

---

[4] Fats (triglycerides) and cholesterol, both good (HDL) and bad (LDL)

[5] CanWest News Service. <u>JAMA</u>, March 7, 2007; 297: 969-977.

Consider the increasing number of patients who undergo weight loss surgery.[6]   Their results are dramatic, but the operations carry a complication rate of over 7%, not including electrolyte and nutritional disturbances that can be life-long. The journal Neurology recently reported that some people, particularly young women, develop neurological symptoms related to vitamin deficiencies once seen only in alcoholics.[7] Unfortunately, many of these people regain a significant portion of their lost weight.   In the case of stomach stapling, the stomach, which was made much smaller by the staples, will eventually stretch back out. Ask any woman who's given birth: the body will compensate and readjust (and stretch).

Some physicians have raised the white flag of surrender. At the April 2007 meeting of the American Association of Endocrinologists it was suggested that gastric bypass surgery could be considered a cure for Type 2 diabetes. However, others admit that using extensive operations to treat a disease that can be managed medically might be ethically controversial.[8]

Maybe drugs are the way to go. In the last few years three of the more popular drugs were removed from the market due to serious complications including heart disease and death.[9] Those still available include orlistat (Xenical), sibutramine (Meridia) and phenteramine (Ionamin).   Similar to the diet programs, the drugs provide only a 5 to 10 pound weight loss

---

[6] There was a 436% increase in bariatric surgeries from 1998 to 2002. In 2003, 103,000 were performed.

[7] Juhasz-Pocsine, K., et al, "Neurologic complications of gastric bypass surgery." Neurology, May 2007; 68: 1843-1850.

[8] Karen Foster-Schubert MD quoted in Medscape Medical News April 13, 2007.

[9] Fenfluramine (Pondimin), dexfenfluramine (Redux) and phenylpropanolamine.

(5%) after one year, with most of the loss in the first six months. Along with these meager results, they are expensive[10] and have multiple side effects including high blood pressure, vitamin deficiencies, and various gastrointestinal problems (abdominal pain, nausea, vomiting and diarrhea).

Regardless, no one can say the government can't be influenced. Convinced with its safety, the FDA will allow orlistat to be sold over the counter as Alli beginning in the summer of 2007. Furthermore, it's in the final stages of approving the use of rimonabant even though the drug is contraindicated for patients with a history of psychiatric disorders—anxiety and depression—common problems in obese patients. Rimonabant is widely used in Europe and is based on manipulating the brain's own marijuana or endocannabinoids.[11] So far there is no miracle drug.

A study comparing caloric restriction versus eating pre-packaged meals found that after 12 weeks both regimens produced similar weight loss (15 pounds) and waist thinning (3 inches). Unfortunately, when the participants were re-measured after 18 months, none of the improvements in body composition or metabolic health continued. Why is it so difficult to maintain long-lasting changes in weight? It was concluded that the reason the results were so impressive in the short term (12 weeks of the diet) was the intensive weekly contact with a dietician.

In January 2002 60 Minutes broadcast a report about the "Lourdes of Lard". In Durham, NC there were three weight loss clinics where obese patients "come to change their ways." The structure and environment provided by the programs is "like a

---

[10] In 2002, the average annual cost per drug was $356.

[11] One of the identified brain peptides has been named anandamide from the Sanskrit ananda or bliss. Ever wonder why someone gets the munchies when "high"?

religious experience."[12]   There were both successes and failures.   The costs of the programs range from $3,000 to $8,000 per month, and the conclusion reached was that there was no quick fix. Any diet will work, but usually only for the time you are on the diet, and especially if you are individually motivated by a health professional or your fellow dieters.

In 1993 the National Weight Control Registry was established.[13]   Membership is reserved for dieters who have lost at least 30 pounds and kept them off for at least one year. The emphasis therefore is on weight maintenance. In the Time Magazine special issue on obesity,[14] it was noted that the Registry lists 5,000 Americans who on average have lost 70 pounds and kept them off at least six years. While there was no consensus about the best diet, the two consistent variables were: limiting what was eaten, and increasing physical activity. Most members limited their calorie intake by decreasing the amount of fat they consumed. The percentages were evenly split as to whether the participants used a formal weight loss program or health care professional versus losing the weight on their own.   The strategies cited most frequently by the participants were:

- 80% ate breakfast daily. In a recent study from by Vanderbilt University, when dieters ate breakfast they lost significantly more weight than those who skipped the morning meal. The proposed mechanisms for this finding included being less hungry throughout the day, less likely to engage in mindless snacking and eating less fat (breakfast foods like oatmeal and fruit contain minimal fat).

---

[12] In May 2007, the BBC had a special on the explosion of weight loss programs in churches in the "Bible Belt".

[13] www.nwcr.ws

[14] "Overcoming Obesity in America" Time Magazine, June 7, 2004.

- Counting calories and eating less fat. On average participants consumed diets which provided about 24% of energy from fat (versus 35% in the average American).[15]
- Exercise daily. The average Registry participant engaged in 60-90 minutes of moderate intensity physical activity daily. Most common activities reported were walking, cycling, aerobics, running or hiking. 28% of the participants used walking as their only exercise.
- 75% weighed themselves daily. Regular monitoring of weight was important to ensure weight maintenance.

In Summary

- It should be obvious by now that the two points that will be hammered home throughout this book are eating less and moving more.
- Make a conscious effort to change, don't be resigned.
- Take action, don't just think about it.
- Pick any diet that you feel comfortable with, but consider it only as one part of a program of weight maintenance.
- The diet you choose should foster weight loss through healthy eating, because you are in it for the long haul.
- You are not alone. Join a weight loss program at work, in your family, church group, or neighborhood.
- Be consistent.

---

[15] Those who follow an Atkins diet obtain 50-75% of calories from fat!

4

Healthy Eating

The meaning of illness is the warning: 'do not continue living as you do.'
Georg Groddeck (1925), founder of
Psychosomatic medicine.

In 1979, Julius Richmond, MD, the US Surgeon General, wrote: "You, the individual, can do more for your own health and well-being than any doctor, any hospital, any drug, or any exotic medical advice." This statement leads us to the Second Commandment: **What's good for your health is good for your diet**. Because this chapter will deal with some basic concepts concerning the food you eat, I will also address the Third Commandment: **To be successful a diet needs to be balanced and offer variety**.

Over 30 years ago the McGovern Commission released a landmark study. After analyzing the current (1977) American diet, it made recommendations that if met were predicted to decrease obesity by 80%, decrease deaths from heart disease by 25% and those from diabetes by 50%. The Commission concluded that longevity would increase by 1% annually, if the following recommendations were met:
- Eat a variety of foods.
- Maintain an ideal weight.

- Avoid too much fat, saturated fat and cholesterol.
- Avoid too much sugar.
- Eat foods with starch and fiber.
- Drink only moderate amounts of alcohol.

Realizing that its recommendations had not been followed and alarmed by the statistics documenting obesity, in 2000 the U.S. Department of Agriculture restated it's objectives, challenging Americans to achieve three basic goals—the ABC's:[1]

Aim for fitness
- Aim for a healthy weight.
- Be physically active each day.

Build a healthy base
- Let the Pyramid guide your food choice.[2]
- Choose a variety of grains daily, especially whole grains.
- Choose a variety of fruits and vegetables daily.
- Keep food safe to eat.

Choose sensibly
- Choose a diet that's low in saturated fat and cholesterol and moderate in total fat.
- Choose beverages and foods to moderate your intake of sugars.
- Choose and prepare foods with less salt.

---

[1] "Dietary Guidelines for Americans, 2000" available at www.usda.gov/cnpp

[2] While 80% of Americans have seen the Food Guide Pyramid, Eric Hentges, director of the USDA's Center for Nutrition Policy and Promotion described one of its shortcomings: "We seem to lack that last step: 'How do I take it and make a behavior change?'" The issue had come up because the government was re-working the pyramid first adopted in 1992. The new recommendations were unveiled in April 2005.

- If you drink alcoholic beverages, do so in moderation.

In 2007 Health Canada released its first update of <u>Canada's Food Guide</u> in 14 years.[3] Like its US counterpart its emphasis is on healthy eating and it has been made more age- and sex-specific than its predecessor. The new guide took over two years of haggling to develop. The most difficult concept to get across is an awareness that in eating—<u>serving size matters</u>.

Diet and longevity

In 1981 Dr. Kenneth Pelletier presented a review of the studies on longevity.[4] Much of the research had been performed on three populations known to have a large number of centenarians: the Vilcabamba in the Ecuadorian Andes, the Hunza in the Himalayas of northern Pakistan, and the Abkhazians in the Caucasus Mountains of Georgia. The most important factor contributing to longevity and optimum health was that "the people are physically active throughout life since they are primarily farmers who labor by hand and walk a great deal in mountainous terrain." It was felt that while hereditary or genetics influenced longevity, their contributions were limited.

Analysis of nutritional and dietary patterns yielded interesting results. The Vilcabambas were exclusively an agricultural community that raised their own vegetables and grains. Their diet provided only 1,200 calories daily, and it was completely vegetarian, with small amounts of protein and fat. The Hunzas ate 1,923 calories daily, and animal protein and fat constituted less than 1% of the daily energy intake. In contrast, the Abkhazians, who raised herds of cows, goats and sheep,

---

[3] <u>www.hc-sc.gc.ca</u> or call 1-800-926-9105, email publications@hc-sc.gc.ca.

[4] <u>Longevity: Fulfilling Our Biological Potential</u>, copyright © 1981 by Kenneth R. Pelletier, Ph.D.

consumed animal products almost daily. They drank milk, ate cheese and yogurt three times a day, and often ate meat. However, two major differences between the diet of the Georgians and our diet today must be highlighted. First, all the milk products were raw, unpasteurized and from goats and sheep as often as from cows. Second, despite the animal products in their diet, the Abkhazians over the age of 50 consumed 1,800 calories daily (400 to 800 calories less than the average sedentary American).

The National Institute of Health is studying the effects of calorie restriction (C.R.)[5]. Ever since the 1930's when a Cornell University nutrition professor discovered that starving rats lived 30% longer, researchers have been intrigued by C.R. During WW I and WW II the shortage of food in the occupied countries of northern Europe led to sharp decreases in the death rates from heart disease, diabetes and cancer.[6] Those rates soared again after the war. While most of us are not obsessive enough to follow a severe C.R. diet, I cite this example to emphasize that eating less has been one of the few lifestyle modifications actually proven to increase lifespan. Perhaps more importantly there is published data suggesting that DNA damage in humans can be decreased by long-term calorie restriction.[7] Is anyone really interested in preserving the human genome?

---

[5] There is a worldwide Calorie Restriction Society. See www.calorierestriction.org

[6] As mentioned previously, contrast to the increases that we see in our children today.

[7] Heilbronn, LK et al, "Effect of 6-month calorie restriction on biomarkers of longevity..." JAMA 2006; 295: 1539-48.

The Food Guide Pyramid

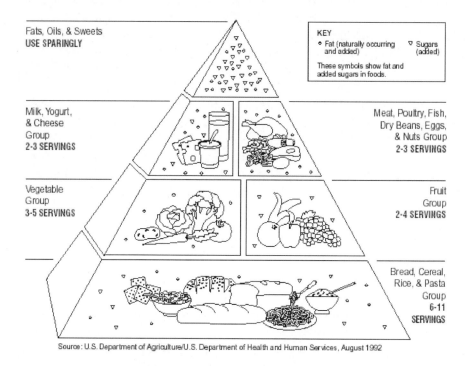

Source: U.S. Department of Agriculture/U.S. Department of Health and Human Services, August 1992

The U.S. government has routinely recommended a balanced diet. The pyramid above was unveiled in 2000. Unfortunately the Consumer Federation noted that the foods that people should eat less of are at the top where they are more easily noticed. Many people believe that what is at the top of the pyramid is most important when just the opposite is true. <u>The concept is that a healthy diet requires a strong base.</u> Notice that the bottom three groups are all plant foods, i.e. grains, fruits and vegetables. The reason for this recommendation is that these foods are low in calories because they are low in fats and simple sugars. They also contain significant amounts of fiber.

Increasing the amount of fiber in the diet of Americans is one of the goals of the USDA recommendations. Fiber comes from plant materials that are not digested easily. One of the primary sources is whole grain. The fiber contained in whole fruits, vegetables and grains increases the rate solid wastes are evacuated. In more "primitive" cultures, the transit time of food through the bowels is 8 to 12 hours. It is not unusual for those of us in more "refined" cultures to have transit times from 3 to 5 days! What do you think happens to the lining of your bowel when it is exposed for such a long time to the toxins contained in waste products? Diverticulosis and colon cancer are commonplace in the modern world.[8] Another benefit of fiber is that it binds cholesterol and other fats in the bowel. Diets high in fiber have been shown to lower the risk of heart disease and stroke by 12%, mainly because of lower cholesterol, especially LDL (low-density lipoprotein).[9]

In April 2005, USDA Secretary Michael Johanns presented the revised nutritional recommendations called "MyPyramid".[10] One of the major short-comings of the 2000 Food Guide Pyramid was the mistaken notion that one size fits all. The revised pyramid offers 12 diet plans ranging from 1,000 calories a day for children to 3,200 calories for athletes. This emphasizes two points:

- The number of servings varies based on the number of calories a person needs to maintain a healthy, stable weight.
- Know thyself!

The new pyramid expands the base from 5 to 9 servings of fruits and vegetables daily to 5 to 13 servings. Also it

---

[8] Colon cancer is the second leading cause of death from cancer.

[9] Containing at least 15.9 grams of fiber daily.

[10] www.mypyramid.gov.

recommends the inclusion of two servings of fish per week, especially those types of fish (e.g. salmon) rich in omega-3 fatty acids which have been shown to reduce the risk of heart disease.

In a recent interview Dr. Kelly Brownell, Director of the Yale Center for Eating and Weight Disorders expressed his concern that <u>the food industry has too much influence on the federal nutrition programs</u>. The government goes along with the food industry in emphasizing exercise and personal responsibility, instead of recommending eating less. He lamented, "I worry that the final pyramid, no matter how good, will have little impact because the government devotes few resources to promoting healthy eating, while the food industry spends massively to encourage people to eat unhealthy food."

Trans fat

Vegetable oils are unsaturated fats and are liquid at room temperature.[11] Saturated fats (such as animal fat, lard) are solid. Unsaturated fats can be made solid by adding hydrogen thereby becoming "partially hydrogenated". The food industry sells us products that have been <u>trans</u>formed by hydrogenation or by heating to a high temperature. Trans fats are found in margarine, vegetable shortening, snacks, crackers, cookies, and in deep-frying fats and oils. They are used by the food industry because they add the characteristic crunch that we all crave, they prolong the shelf life of fat and products with fat, and they reduce cost. Research has shown that the amount of trans fat produced in cooking is dependent on the method used (more in deep-frying, less when pan frying), the type of oil (least from olive oil, most from sunflower) and the freshness of

---

[11] Mono-unsaturated such as olive oil, and poly-unsaturated such as canola oil.

the oil (increase with older oil—think—deep fryer at a fast food chain).[12]

In 1990 studies conclusively demonstrated that <u>trans fat increases bad cholesterol (LDL) and decreases good cholesterol</u>. It took another 12 years before the National Institute of Medicine concluded that there is <u>no safe level of trans fat in the diet</u>! They are easily taken up by fat cells and thereby make weight loss more difficult. They decrease testosterone, disrupt immune function and raise insulin levels. <u>For every 2% (4-5 grams or the amount in one donut) increase in trans fat consumption there is a doubling of the risk for heart disease</u>.

After first being proposed in 1994 by the Center for Science in the Public Interest (CSPI),[13] the FDA (even though it knew about the issue in the 1980's) finally mandated that as of January 1, 2006 trans fat must be included on the Nutrition Facts label. Resistance to this effort was strong because trans fats are a multi-billion dollar industry, and most believe that inclusion of trans fat on the label will be the death knell for the industry.

Many of the companies that hydrogenate are represented by the Institute of Shortening and Edible Oils, which was lobbying the government to prevent the release of the bad news concerning trans fat.[14] Even though evidence began surfacing

---

[12] A <u>New England Journal of Medicine</u> correspondence (April 13, 2006; Vol. 295: 1650-52) determined that the content of trans fat in fast food varied according to country. A large fries and chicken nugget combo in <u>New York City had 10.2 grams vs. 0.33 grams in Denmark</u> which banned trans fat, and 3 grams in Spain, Russia and the Czech Republic.

[13] http://transfreeamerica.org or www.cspinet.org

[14] In 1995 ISEO President Robert Reeves said in an interview about the safety of trans fats on the BBC: "I'm confident they're safe in the diet at their current levels of consumption."

in the late 1960's, industry scientists refuted the efforts of researchers to make this news public, and in fact scorned the research as "bad science".

It takes the federal government a long time to get out from under industry lobbyists like the American Soybean Association.[15] To emphasize that this is a North American problem, the Heart and Stroke Foundation of Canada reported in 2007 that Canadians are the biggest consumers of trans fats in the world—ingesting 4.9 grams of the toxin every day.

One last note of caution must be raised. I've recently noticed the label "0 grams of trans fat" on many foods like cookies and potato chips. In this way the products are marketed as safe and healthy, or at least non-toxic. Unfortunately beware that they still may contain loads of fat. Applaud the governments for the requirement to label levels of trans fat, but never underestimate the ingenuity of salesmen trying to deceive us.

In Summary

While it may be difficult to completely trust what the nutritional authorities recommend, there are some constants to a healthy diet:

- Eat less. Be aware of serving size.
- Eat a variety of foods.
- The foundation of any healthy diet is fresh fruits, vegetables and whole grains—the broad base of the Food Guide Pyramid.
- Avoid all trans fat—think crispy, deep-fried, processed foods.
- Know what you are eating—beware and be aware!
- Know thyself—what others can eat (regardless of what the "experts" say) may not be what you should eat.

---

[15] Soybean oil accounts for 85% of trans fats.

5

The Case against Processed Foods

The next Commandment is: **The best diet would be simple: low cost, readily available foods that are easy to prepare**. Due to the time constraints that we place ourselves under, Americans have chosen the fast-food route. There just isn't enough time to prepare a home cooked meal. As mentioned previously this problem is rampant in Western societies, yet people in other countries make it a point to retain this connection with their past. Food is culture, not a commodity. In the rush to develop and provide food for Americans, the food industry has changed our palette.

When I lived in upstate New York I remember picking an apple from an old tree on my property. It was small and gnarled, but when I bit into the speckled skin, its texture and tart taste exploded in my mouth. As I chewed, the juice became sweeter and added complexity to the flavor. Most apples today have been picked green, left in cold storage for long periods of time, and are flavorless. I offered one of my apples to a friend whose mouth initially puckered due to the tartness, but eventually widened in a grin of appreciation for this new (or was it only forgotten?) experience.

There has been a movement towards growing giant, beautiful, premium-priced fruits and vegetables.[1] A recent article in Gourmet marveled that apples, plums, pears, oranges and strawberries are up to twice as big as they were 25 years ago. Large supermarket chains figured that it's cheaper to harvest, sort and stock a few giant fruits rather than many smaller ones. However, quality tends to suffer as size increases, as one grower noted: "For every apple there's only so much flavor, and if you grow it larger, you dilute it."[2] Many of us realize that our store-bought foods are deficient, as evidenced by the numerous "farmer's markets" that have sprouted up in our cities and towns.[3]

In most of the world almost every town has a local produce market that is open two to three days per week. In Europe, this is a tradition that goes back before the Middle Ages. What is their attraction? While supermarkets offer a measure of convenience, the local markets offer freshness, vitality and uniqueness that cannot be duplicated in processed, brightly packaged, long shelf-lived foods. A few years back, on a trip to the coast of France, I stopped at a local farmer's market and was handed a few grapes to sample by the grower. He beamed proudly when I tasted their incredible, wine-like flavor and nodded in appreciation.

When I walked through a Bon Marche supermarket in Paris, I couldn't find many canned foods. There were huge fresh fish, produce and bakery sections. There also were isles dedicated to foods from around the world. I was shocked when I stood before the "North American" isle. On its shelves were stocked such staples as peanut butter (processed with salt and corn

---

[1] Sounds like Hollywood, doesn't it?

[2] Stephen Wood quoted in Gourmet, July 2005, page 38.

[3] In 1994 there were 1,755 farmer's markets; in August 2004 there were 3,137.

sweetener) and cranberry sauce. Also included in the foods representing this side of the Atlantic were boxed pancake mix, pancake syrup with maple flavoring, Marshmallow Fluff, strawberry milk flavoring and (I'm not making this up) cocktail wieners.

Not long ago a large supermarket moved into town. Its shelves were full of different brands of coffee, cereal, canned goods and even pet food. As time passed, the store stopped carrying such a large variety. I assumed that this was done because these products weren't selling, however, sometimes I wonder whether the store is just manipulating my choices, and ultimately my taste.

Sadly it seems the European Union is changing the food supplies of its member countries to be more like that of North America. On a trip this year I stopped in a market and purchased some big, beautiful grapes from South Africa. Like the fruit we buy from South America, they look great, but they have no taste. Transport your food 10,000 miles and guess what you get—bland, magically preserved, unsatisfying food!

The USDA and FDA have taken it upon themselves to provide safe food. The goal of these agencies is to insure that no food is dangerous to anyone. Look how the airlines and school districts have placed the peanut alongside illegal drugs, or even terrorists, as a life threatening menace. Perhaps the peanut will go the way of raw milk and cheese, and be banished from our food supply all together. Too bad most of the evidence concerning the dangers of these living foods points to problems with packaging and delivery.

The contamination of our meat supply with E. coli and Salmonella (contained in feces) is related to the filthy conditions of over-crowded feedlots used in factory farming. Goodbye, medium rare hamburgers! If E. coli exists mainly in the stool of animals, how does it get into washed pre-packaged lettuce? Hmm!

The recent mad-cow scare can be traced to the ingestion of infected neural tissue[4] by the animals. In other words, the cows eat the brains of other infected cows. Thirty years ago in medical school I learned about kuru, which was a degenerative brain disease (strikingly similar to mad-cow) found only in cannibal societies that ate the brains of their victims. What do they say about the past: those who forget it are bound to repeat it?

It is interesting how Americans have actually heeded the government's recommendations to eat more vegetables. Since 1920 we've doubled our intake of vegetables, but now we eat more processed vegetables than we used to eat vegetables in total. The percentage of fresh to processed vegetables has dropped from 70% to 43%. A similar pattern has occurred in fruit consumption. While nutritionists proudly boast of a 45% increase in fruit consumption since 1920, the percentage of fresh fruit has dropped from 83% to 33%. Why should these statistics be a problem? Remember, French fries are the number one vegetable and also that ketchup is considered a vegetable.[5] Consider that an equivalent amount of processed to fresh fruit has over twice the calories and half the fiber.[6] North Americans spend 90% of their food dollar on processed foods. They provide us with a huge variety of inexpensive food, but it doesn't come cheap.

Food processing adds sugar and salt and removes many of the life-giving properties of the natural food including fiber, vitamins and minerals. The FDA allows the processors to add a witch's brew of artificial chemicals to stabilize, preserve, color and flavor the food. Most of these additives are given the classification GRAS (Generally Regarded As Safe). Doesn't

---

[4] Brain and spinal cord.

[5] 81% of the calories in ketchup come from corn syrup.

[6] Again, because of the addition of simple sugars.

sound like our own government is totally convinced! In the recent lawsuit brought against it by some obese children, McDonald's own lawyers were quoted that it was "a matter of common knowledge that any processing that its foods undergo serves to make them more harmful than unprocessed foods."

The goal of the food processor is to sell more food, so you will eat more food, et cetera. Food processing makes it more uniform and consistent (reliable) and makes it last longer (for transport and shelf-life), but it also adds calories and devitalizes the food. Unlike my home-grown apple, many store-bought foods no longer satisfy the taste buds. Whatever happened to the juicy red tomato? Do not underestimate smell, color, taste and texture and their influence on satiation. In other words, the more satisfying the food, the more satiated we feel, and in the end, the less we need to eat.

When rats are given the choice between white flour (from which the bran and germ have been removed) and whole wheat flour, they eat the more complete and healthy food. A Tufts University study of 3,000 people found that those who ate three daily servings of whole grains[7] were 33% less likely to develop metabolic syndrome[8] than those eating less than one serving per week.

It takes a little extra effort to buy and utilize whole foods. However, some of the joys of eating are in the acquisition and preparation. In the center of Rome, there is a piazza called the Campo di Fiore. Every day there is a farmer's market that sells brightly colored fruits and vegetables along with fish and meat. The people walk through the market on their way to and from work, and stop to buy what is fresh that day. You see them heading back to their homes with bags to prepare the noon or evening meals. Can you imagine Americans shopping every

---

[7] The average American eats less than one serving of whole grains daily.

[8] Diabetes + hypertension + high blood cholesterol + abdominal obesity.

day? We live a different life and because of how we live we are relegated to buying processed foods, overeating and growing ever larger.

I realize that some of us don't have the time or the income to spend on totally changing our diet, but to pack a lunch with whole wheat bread and fresh meat or cheese or peanut butter, along with a piece of fruit would be a start in the right direction. Whole grain cereal, yogurt or fresh eggs and toast would be an improvement over most breakfasts. Loose leaf green salad with home-made dressing (olive oil and vinegar), followed by a baked potato and a piece of fresh meat or fish would be a simple and inexpensive finish to a nutritious day's meals. A little effort goes a long way.

Keep it simple

Perhaps you've heard the expression "the wisdom of the body". I hate to tell you this, but the body really isn't very smart. It knows some very basic, stereotypical ways of doing things, and it will adhere to these ways. Take the example of our emotional reaction to external events. A prehistoric man was sitting by the river's edge when he heard something rustling in the tall grass behind him. The hair on his back bristled as his nostrils and pupils dilated. His heart pounded and his muscles became taut as he slowly picked up his spear and turned towards the noise. Suddenly from the grass emerged a saber-tooth tiger. The man cocked his arm and flung the spear at the hungry animal. He did not wait to see whether the spear hit the mark but instead leaped into the river to swim away.

Fast-forward to the present day. You are sitting at your desk in front of the computer when your boss, who always seems to be on your back, steps into your cubicle. She confronts you about a report that besides being late is not what she wanted. You take a deep breath trying to relax the tightening muscles in your neck but as you do so your nostrils and pupils dilate. Your blood pressure goes up and your fists tighten.   Then she warns, "I expect the corrected report on my desk by the end of the day!" Knowing that you've got a date for dinner, just as you pick up your spear—I mean pen—to thrust at her, you clench your teeth, swallow hard and reply meekly, "Sure thing." Your body reacted to a stressful situation just like that of your prehistoric ancestor, only in today's world you have to internalize your distress. This response is called "fight or flight," yet you can do neither! Stress creates a toxic environment in which damage accumulates. We haven't changed much over time. How's that for wisdom?

It amazes me when I eat out or read the ingredients of many nouveau, cutting edge recipes. Your digestive system secretes enzymes to break down what you eat so that the nutrients of the diet can be absorbed. The last chapter advocated variety in your diet. However, I do not believe you should combine every food type in one recipe or even in one meal. This mistaken belief often borders on abuse at highly-acclaimed restaurants. Food critics have gone "Hollywood": praising appearance and stylized production over taste. Too often you consume the ego of some famous chef who serves alchemical concoctions that don't make much sense. How's the stomach going to handle foie gras, olives, ginger, butter and cream served over a bed of pumpkin risotto? Confusion reigns supreme.

<u>The body has to have some idea what it's trying to digest, i.e. protein, fat, dairy, wheat or fruit. It has to make sense</u>. Read the ingredients list on any processed food. What's the body supposed to do with chicken pieces, modified food starch, encapsulated salt, casein, partially hydrogenated soybean oil, sodium citrate, artificial flavors, yellow #5 and #6, sodium erythorbate, ethoxylated mono- and di-glycerides, chicken fat and tricalcium phosphate?

As we try to simplify our diet we have to go back to basics. Many nutritionists consider the diet eaten by those living around the Mediterranean Sea to be one of the healthiest. It is plant based, and low in saturated fat with olive oil being the principle fat.[9]   Bread, pasta, rice, couscous and polenta (cornmeal) are common. Fish is eaten as often as meat. What jumps out at you most when you eat in the Mediterranean countries is that the emphasis is on freshness of ingredients and simplicity of preparation. Like Picasso who composed his paintings with the fewest number of elements, the cook needs only the basics to make great art. Grilled fish basted with olive oil and salt. Spinach lightly cooked with butter and lemon. Potatoes baked in the oven with olive oil and rosemary. Real food, cooked simply!

Faux food

Part of the problem with processed foods is that they no longer bear much resemblance to when they were in their natural state. Millions of years of evolution are thrown out the window when we consume artificial foods. This brings us to the next Commandment: **Don't try to fake out your body! Eat real food.**   Maybe if we were able to recognize what we were eating, our bodies would be much more satisfied. You can't fool Mother Nature.

Besides the inclusion of various chemicals to enhance and preserve processed foods, another problem with the industrialization of our food supply is the development of artificial flavors and foods.[10] Faux foods. What is a fruit roll-up? How about those chips in a can? Margarine is not used much in Europe with most people preferring butter. Can saccharine or aspartame actually be less harmful for you than

---

[9] Olive oil, along with canola and peanut oils are high in monounsaturated fat. Other similar foods include avocados, olives, most nuts including peanuts, almonds and pecans, and nut butters including tahini or sesame paste.

[10] I am not even mentioning bioengineered foods which are another whole discussion. In 1994 the FDA had approved 1 bioengineered food, today there are 54 different foods.

the reasonable use of sugar, or better yet, molasses or honey? How do they transform corn or wheat or oats into Captain Crunch, Fruit loops or Corn Pops?[11] I was amazed at <u>how similar the ingredients for the dog treat Snausages, were to those contained in Hot Pockets</u>. In an article about the "Naked chef" turned activist Jamie Oliver, the author wrote:

> To shock the older children into nutritional awareness, he tossed a chicken carcass into a blender along with bits of skin, fat and bread crumbs, whizzed it around, and showed off the result: stomach-turning mush that, when shaped and cooked, could pass for the nuggets they had been eating.[12]

When you eat faux food you could be eating anything!

It's not just a matter of obesity—it's about health. It has taken time for Britain's school children to accept the foods offered by the "Naked Chief". However, not only have they come to like the healthier, more nutritious offerings mandated by the government's $535 million program, other benefits have begun to surface. Parents have reported that their children are behaving better at home, and in school their teachers have seen improvements in concentration and academic achievement.

Food in its natural state contains many of the enzymes and cofactors necessary for rapid absorption and assimilation of nutrients. Faux foods contain none of these aids to digestion forcing our bodies to overwork. The food sits in our stomachs

---

[11] I remember as a kid that Corn Pops were called Sugar Pops. I assume that the name had to be changed because sugar fell out of favor. It's all in the marketing.

[12] Sarah Lyall, <u>International Herald Tribune</u>, April 23, 2005.

for long periods of time, increasing the pressure on the gastro-esophageal valve which fails over time—leading to reflux disease.[13] Do you think it's a coincidence that one of the top three advertised drugs (along with cholesterol lowering statins and erectile dysfunction meds) is for gastroesophageal reflux disease (GERD)? The liver, gall bladder and pancreas are also severely overstressed by the confusing elements presented to the small bowel for digestion. Because they churn out enzymes trying to deal with the overload, eventually they are bound to fail.

There has always been controversy concerning the safety of food additives and substitutes. The artificial sweetener market is incredibly lucrative and has had its share of detractors. Cyclamates were banned in the early 1970's because they were linked to bladder cancer, yet they have recently begun to be investigated again. Saccharine has been around for over 100 years and has fallen in and out of favor. Aspartame is known to be broken down into the toxic by-products methanol, formaldehyde and formic acid. In the last 20 years there have been over 400 studies addressing the safety of aspartame. 100% of those funded by the drug company that produces aspartame found it absolutely safe. Yet every one of those performed by independent investigators brought up questions of its safety. The FDA has stood by the research that considers aspartame safe, but remember that it took 35 years for the agency to mandate caution in the area of trans fat. In a recent study from Purdue University rats given artificial sweeteners ate three times more calories than rats given sugar.[14] Researchers hypothesize that the artificial sweeteners interfere with the body's ability to regulate food and calorie consumption based on the perception of sweetness. Could

---

[13] Obese abdomens also put more pressure on the valve, increasing the chance of hiatal hernia.

[14] "A Pavlovian approach to the problem of obesity", Int J Obesity, July 2004.

artificial sweeteners actually be making us fatter? The bottom line: it is best to avoid faux foods.

As an emergency physician I see pretty sick people every day. I have always believed that the way back to health is to have them understand how they contribute to their own illness. I have stressed this not to point fingers and make them feel guilty, but to empower them and offer them the way out—to take control of their health. Medical therapies can be very effective, but your natural healing powers are even more important. Quite often when I see a very old (over 90-95 years) patient, she is accompanied by a relative who proudly states: "She's on no medicine and doesn't even see a doctor!" I laugh and praise the accomplishment, yet it's obvious to me that the reason they've lived so long is that they <u>are</u> healthy and have healthy habits. The nutritionist Paavo Airola noted that you never see obese centenarians.[15] They also tend not be over-medicated and over-doctored. Unfortunately we have been led to believe that medications are the cure-all. "Doctor, you must have something for my..."

Once again it comes down to culture and education. There are an incredible number of healthy octogenarians living on the island of Okinawa. They eat a traditional diet composed of vegetable, soy products, fruit and sea vegetables. Most importantly they're passing their healthy habits on to their great grand-children. Freelance journalist Eugenie Francoeur wrote about her visit to a primary school. A teacher offered:

> "From a young age, the students are taught the importance of food and all the respect we should give it." The children were able to list the foods to eat to avoid high blood pressure, cholesterol, constipation and heart disease. Before leaving, I

---

[15] <u>How to Get Well</u>. Health Plus Publishers, Sherwood, Oregon © 1974.

> try to find out if there are any cases of
> hyperactive children there.   Surprised by my
> question, the teacher says the school has never
> had any cases of hyperactivity. I want to make
> sure the head teacher understands my question
> correctly, so I rephrase it. "Are there any children
> here who take Ritalin or other medication to calm
> the turbulent ones and help them improve their
> concentration?" With a horrified look on her face,
> she replies: "Of course not. <u>Why would we do
> that to our children</u>?"[16]

Pharmaceutical companies are incredibly influential on our
culture through their advantageous manipulation of government
policy. The more drugs they sell the more profit they make and
the more their stock goes up. In 2002, the combined profits of
the ten drug companies in the Fortune 500 were larger than
those of the other 490 companies combined![17] In 2003 the
drug company trade organization, Pharmaceutical Research
and Manufacturers of America (PhRMA), spent $126.3 million
to lobby Congress and state legislatures.   Money buys
influence. There really is no incentive for them to get or to
keep people healthy. The fact is <u>the drug companies depend
on sick people for their very survival</u>.

We are clamoring for help in paying for prescription drugs. We
spend exorbitant amounts of money on healthcare, yet we
refuse to pay for organic foods that have been certified free of
pesticides, fertilizers and additives.[18] A recent government
study found that many people complain that the cost of fresh

---

[16] <u>The Globe and Mail</u> April 29, 2006, page F9.

[17] $35.5 billion to $33.7 billion. <u>Public Citizen Congress Watch</u>, June 2003
(www.citizen.org/documents/Pharma_Report.pdf).

[18] For a summary on organic foods and the toxins in today's food supply see
www.medicalnewstoday.com/medicalnews.php?newsid=10587.

fruits and vegetables prevents them from eating more produce. Yet the same USDA survey found that consumers could get the daily recommended servings of fruits and vegetable for just 64 cents.

Organic produce is just pennies more and becoming more readily available.[19] In 1994 there were 4,050 certified organic farms, today there are 11,998. Most high-end restaurants use organic fruits and vegetables because of their taste and consistency. There is data coming out of Italy (where soil management, not hyper-fertilization, is a priority) that shows fruits grown organically are higher in minerals, vitamins and anti-oxidants. We spend less than 10% of our personal income for food while healthcare accounts for over 16% of the GNP. It seems like our priorities are out of whack! I realize that it's not quite this simple, but wouldn't you rather spend time and money eating a good healthy meal than be in the doctor's office waiting for an expensive and possibly harmful drug? Your food should be your medicine.

Perhaps just as important as eating organic foods is buying locally raised and grown foods. When I was a kid I couldn't wait for June's strawberry season, fresh corn on the cob in August and apples in the fall. Today we don't flinch when we see perfect looking (not tasting) tomatoes in January. Former Columbia University professor of nutrition Joan Gussow has complained that shipping a strawberry from California to New York requires 435 calories of fossil fuel but provides the eater with only 5 calories of nutrition. As the author of This Organic Life she has acknowledged, "People need to know that they may have fewer choices if they eat locally and by the seasons." Forget about Al Gore, the G8 and the Kyoto Protocol. Turn off your television with its food and drug ads. Walk past your doctor's office by simplifying your life. Your waistline, pocketbook and the earth itself will smile back in appreciation.

---

[19] Even Wal-Mart is getting into the business by offering organic foods at only a 10% premium over its regular produce.

In Summary

- Your food is your medicine.[20]
- Eat real, fresh, whole foods.
- Give your body time to digest.
- Read the label. Avoid faux foods. Minimize use of processed foods.
- Buy organic when and if possible.
- Know your supplier. Buy local. Visit farmer's markets. Better yet grow your own.
- Keep your choices, ingredients and combinations simple.
- "Freshness, locality and seasonability."[21]
- To every thing there is a season, and a time to every purpose under the heaven: a time to be born, and a time to die; a time to plant, and a time to pluck up that which is planted.[22]

---

[20] "Let food be your medicine and medicine be your food," Hippocrates (c.460-400 BCE).

[21] Alice Waters.

[22] Ecclesiastes 3: 1-2.

6

Knowledge is Power

The experientially empty person, lacking these directives from within, these voices of the real self, must turn to outer cues for guidance, for instance eating when the clock tells him to, rather than obeying his appetite (he has none). He guides himself by clocks, rules, calendars, schedules, agenda, and by hints and cues from other people.[1]

A Time Magazine/ABC News poll found that 74% of respondents wanted warning labels on high-fat and high-sugar foods and 61% would support a law requiring restaurants to include dietary information such as calories and types of fat on menus. 53% believed that the Federal government was doing too little to address the problem of obesity.[2]

---

[1] Abraham Maslow, The Farther Reaches of Human Nature, p. 32. Viking Penguin Inc, New York, NY, 1971.

[2] Conducted May 10-16 and quoted in Time Magazine, June 7, 2004.

This brings us to the next Commandment: **Knowledge is power. Know what you eat.** Perhaps this is the most obvious commandment, but it may also be the most subtle, for knowledge includes awareness of both the internal and external cues.

I was driving down the expressway the other day when a young woman zipped by me. After my initial displeasure with being passed, I became concerned with how erratic she was driving as she began to swerve into my lane. At first I thought she was on a cell phone, until I noticed that she was chowing down on some sort of sandwich. Insurance specialists have noted that eating in cars may be just as dangerous as using cell phones.[3] Forget about safety, how can anyone driving a car be aware of what he or she is eating? In the "60 Minutes" piece on the weight loss clinics in Durham, North Carolina, a 400 pound man said that he would call his wife on his way home from work and ask what she was having for dinner. Assuming she would not make enough, he would then stop at the local fast-food joint and order take-out. It's impossible to read the internal cues that your body gives off when you are performing multiple tasks at the same time that you are eating. Recall that 67% of office workers eat lunch at their desks!

In a recent survey conducted by Baylor College of Medicine researchers found that more than 42% of dinners at home were eaten while watching TV. Even more damning was that 50% of overweight children ate dinner in front of the television. Unfortunately like Pavlov's dog that had been conditioned to associate the ringing of a bell with dinner causing his mouth to water, we are conditioned to associate watching TV with eating![4]

---

[3] Michael Haggerty, NPR "Talk of the Nation", August 8, 2002.

[4] Remember that the body really isn't very wise.

What's worse is that most of the food eaten in front of the TV is high calorie and high fat snack foods. What do we eat in a movie theater? Either a gigantic tub of buttery salty popcorn, nachos with some sort of liquid cheese-flavored goo or a candy bar, and not those little ones we used to eat, but some sort of gargantuan candy mutant! Afterwards you wash it all down with a monstrous soda. In counseling patients, I keep referencing to a recent commercial that shows a guy running through the streets cradling a bucket of chicken, when he reaches home he asks, "Is it still half-time?" The next thing you know someone is at the door handing him 64 ounces of soda-pop—that's 900 calories of flavored corn syrup! Beware and be aware.

The myth of security

A physician friend of mine told me that when his family was in Germany the only place that his kids felt comfortable—where they could get a good (read trusty) meal—was at McDonald's. I actually appreciate fast-food restaurants. I have often joked that McDonald's is the gas station of the new millennium. As a kid, when my family traveled, we trusted gas stations to provide comfort facilities. Today, the fast food chains have taken over that role.

I have been told that the reason people eat where or how they do is because they know what the meal will be like. In another recent article, the regional manager of a national chain restaurant summed up the feeling of most of his customers: "Going out to eat is risky. You never know what you're going to get."[5] What a sad commentary if that's the reason for the success of the food industry. If we have reduced food to sameness and security, it's not even worth eating. Variety is the spice of life. Part of the joy of travel, or even eating at the home of friends, is that you will experience something

---

[5] Rebecca Skloot, New York Times Magazine, October 17, 2004.

different—something outside yourself that may expand your world. I've heard it said that you must be able to think a new thought in order to change your thinking. Unfortunately in a recent survey 33% of obese respondents thought that their weight was just right. Even 5% of those who were morbidly obese believed that they were just the right size.

Psychologists have long recognized our emotional connection to food. "Hunger, as a characteristic expression of the instinct of self-preservation, is without a doubt one of the primary and most important factors in influencing behavior."[6] Unfortunately eating is often used as a means to cope with the stress of daily life and to assuage negative emotional states such as depression, anxiety, boredom, or loneliness.[7] Many of us become distressed because we fear not getting enough food. Realize however, that our minds crave food even more than our bodies.[8]

<u>Food gives us comfort because we have allowed and even encouraged our bodies to attach to it</u>. Putting it another way, without food we become agitated. The national chains know this and have conditioned us to believe that our agitation can be soothed most readily by eating in their restaurants. I recognize the sign out front and I feel safe once again, for I can count on the meal to be what I expect. Understand that the restaurants are selling security. They are not really giving your body what it needs, only what your mind believes it needs—a safe haven in an ocean of confusion and agitation.

---

[6] Karl Jung, "Psychological Factors in Human Behavior," <u>The Structure and Dynamics of the Psyche</u>, Collected Works, par. 237.

[7] Ganley RM, "Emotion and eating in obesity," <u>Int J Eating Disorders</u>: 8, p. 343-361; 1989.

[8] This helps to partially explain anorexia nervosa. Starvation is the way that the patient can take control of her environment, and in the end the strength of her mind starves the body.

Try the following exercise:

1. When you sit down to eat be aware of what you are eating. Know the ingredients, how they were prepared and as much as possible, where they came from.
2. Take a moment or two to appreciate the look, smell and feel of the food.
3. Chew every bite slowly to fully enjoy its taste and texture. Is there an aftertaste?
4. Swallow each mouthful before taking another. This will slow down the meal.
5. Pause between courses. Let your mind catch up to the body's internal cues.
6. Concentration should require some effort, but it should not cause tension, restriction or guilt.
7. Enjoy the company of others but don't let them distract you from becoming aware of your body's needs or desires.

Repeat the exercise as often as possible. In time you will slow down your eating and appreciate the food more. Some other things may happen. You will become more aware of the food's freshness and if you are eating processed foods, you may begin to taste the chemicals that they contain. You won't eat as much because you will begin to read the internal cues. Try to become aware of your realistic needs and then strive to attain them, but try not to reach beyond them.

In a national survey of 1500 Canadian adults conducted by Leger marketing, 31% said they consciously consume a food or drink they know will give them problems like heartburn, cramps, gas or diarrhea at least once a week. 8% admitted to making these choices daily! Women were more likely than men to ignore these internal cues.[9] Where's the pleasure in making yourself uncomfortable or sick?

---

[9] CanWest News Service, quoted in the National Post, March 6, 2007.

One of the reasons that many of us overeat on holidays is that the distraction of our fellow diners prevents us from reading our internal cues. What mother hasn't complained after cooking all day that the holiday meal is devoured in minutes? Research has shown that individuals at a group meal take their cues from a "pacesetter". If the pacesetter eats slowly, the rest of the group will follow. Speed up—they all eat quickly. The group will also respond to how much she eats: eat one cookie—it's one cookie each, gobble down handfuls of chips... Enjoy yourself, but slow down. Amazingly everyone else will too![10]

Another exercise is to ask yourself the seven rays of discernment:

1. *What* food am I eating?
2. *When* am I eating?
3. *Why* am I eating?
4. *Where* am I eating?
5. *Who* is eating?
6. *How* am I eating?
7. *Which* meal am I eating?

Make an affirmation to become more aware of what you eat. You may not completely stop eating bad things, but hopefully you'll stop feeding yourself mindlessly. Take time to study your habits. Don't become angry when you falter because that will only increase the mind's agitation—to be once again soothed by eating more! Remember, all diets fail.

Calories are important

It seems as if everybody today is counting carbs, fats or points. A recent report from the USDA Center for Nutrition Policy and Promotion recommended: "To stem the obesity epidemic, most

---

[10] Unfortunately moms this may fall on your shoulders. You probably buy the food, cook it and set it out. You may have to be your family's pacesetter as well.

Americans need to reduce the amount of calories they consume. When it comes to weight control, calories do count—not the proportions of carbohydrate, fat and protein in the diet." Besides adding trans fat, the FDA is considering revising the Nutrition Facts Label by making the word "calories" larger and bolder. We've gotten away from the fact that every person has a level of calories that will maintain the proper weight. Obviously when we consume more than our maintenance level, we gain weight, less and we lose.

The Basal Metabolic Rate (BMR) is the number of calories that your body needs for daily functioning (i.e. digestion, circulation and breathing). Knowing your BMR should help you to establish your maintenance caloric intake. There are many elaborate formulas to calculate your BMR. Some people read books, go to health clubs, even websites[11] but most experts admit that any method brings with it a 10% margin of error. An easy method to calculate your BMR is as follows:

- Multiply your weight in pounds X 11 = BMR
- If sedentary, daily caloric requirement = BMR X 1.2
- Light activity, daily requirement = BMR X 1.3-1.4
- Moderate activity, daily requirement = BMR X 1.5
- If very active, daily requirement = BMR X 1.6-1.7
- Extremely active, daily requirement = BMR X 2-2.4

Once you know your BMR you can figure out how much weight you can lose or gain by knowing how many calories you eat in a day. <u>One pound of weight will be added or lost with every addition or deficit of 3600 calories</u>. Knowing this information makes it easier to see the reason for the increase of obesity.

Drinking one 12 ounce can of soda, juice, beer or milk more than we need each day for a year will result in a weight gain of 15 pounds.[12] Do that for five years and you've added 75

---

[11] www.kidsnutrition.org/caloriesneed.html.

pounds! Similarly, any diet that claims you will lose 10 pounds in a week is banking on losing water weight, because it would be physiologically impossible to accumulate a deficit of 36,000 calories in a week unless you ate nothing, and your BMR was 5143 calories.[13]   One gallon of water weighs over 7 pounds. Therefore, to lose what most diets in magazines claim requires 1-2 gallons of water weight loss in a short period of time. Doesn't sound very healthy, does it?

To count calories you need the following:

- A reliable source of caloric food values.
- Read the Nutrition Facts Label.
- A way to measure your food and/or a convenient way to estimate portion size.
- Don't be obsessive about it. It's got to be fun to do. Everything that you are counting, measuring and researching is only an estimate.

A convenient way to estimate portion size is to look at your own hand:

- 1 thumb print = 1 teaspoon
- 2 thumb prints = 1 tablespoon
- Palm of hand = 4 ounces (i.e. fish or meat)
- Palm with fingers and thumb = 8 ounces (1/2 pound)
- Fist = 1 cup

Obviously we all have different size hands, but it's all relative anyway. A large handed man would have a higher BMR and need more calories.

---

[12] 150 calories X 365 days = 54,750 surplus calories / 3600 calories per pound = 15.2 pounds.

[13] 36,000 calories / 7 days = 5143 calories per day.

What about carbohydrates?

Carbohydrates are the main source of energy for the body. When proteins or fats are used for energy (as in starvation) they must first be broken down and converted to the end product of carbohydrate metabolism. Carbohydrates actually decrease the protein requirement in the diet, because the body does not have to break down protein for energy.[14]

There are two large groups of carbohydrates: starches or complex carbohydrates (polysaccharides) and simple sugars (mono- and disaccharides). Carbohydrates can also be classified as either naturally occurring or refined. Naturally occurring carbohydrates include the simple sugars in fruit or milk,[15] and the starches contained in pasta, rice and potato. Naturally occurring carbohydrates are bound together with fiber—another important dietary component. Refined carbohydrates are added to processed foods for taste, preservation and consistency. As already mentioned, usually they are in the form of simple sugars,[16] and they serve to increase the caloric content while removing fiber and beneficial nutrients.

The average American eats his weight in sugar every year. I am talking about sugar as purified sugar cane—not complex carbohydrate. Candy, soda, juice and sugary desserts are not the same thing as rice, potatoes and macaroni. Diabetics are commonly prescribed a diet that is high in complex carbohydrate (especially the low glycemic index type) and low in fat. This type of diet can improve insulin secretion and therefore stabilize blood sugar levels. Studies have also shown that complex carbohydrates will lower blood lipids and

---

[14] Protein-sparing effect.

[15] Glucose, fructose and lactose.

[16] Sucrose and high-fructose corn syrup.

decrease atherosclerosis (heart disease and hardening of the arteries). Eating a diet high in simple sugar results in high blood sugar level and forces the body to secrete insulin to drive the level back down. The result may be hypoglycemia (low blood sugar) that sends a signal back to the brain that you need more sugar. We get tricked into a cycle of highs and lows.

Within the brain, carbohydrates release serotonin which is the neurotransmitter responsible for peace and pleasure. Serotonin induces sleep. Interestingly, the newest antidepressants are serotonin blockers. Could it be that one of the attractions of the low carb diets is their effect on the brain? That is, there would be lower levels of serotonin in the brain when a strict low carb diet is followed: less serotonin = less calm = less fatigue (?), more stimulation in a time of hyper-stimulation. <u>Dieting Americans on speed</u>. Perhaps the low carb craze is actually just an addiction—cocaine, caffeine, low carb! Realize that addictions don't make any sense, they aren't logical. Watch someone destroy their life through an addiction and you ask yourself: can't they see it? Trying to separate out the nutrients of your diet by replacing natural whole foods with low carb faux foods doesn't make any sense either.

Don't eat out

When you eat out, it is very difficult to lose or control your weight. In <u>USA Today</u> the author wrote: "Even in an age of better-educated dining, decadence still beats out decorum when most Americans eat out."[17] I am not advocating that you totally avoid restaurants. However, the way to be most aware of what you are eating is to purchase, prepare and eat your own food. Many restaurants are starting to make the nutrient lists of their recipes available, especially the fast food and national chain restaurants. Consult them.

---

[17] "Restaurant sales climb with bad-for-you food" <u>USA Today</u>, May 13, 2005.

Beware and be aware. The foods served in restaurants tend to be nutrient dense and the servings are too large. Use the method I gave you to estimate portion sizes the next time you are in a restaurant. Notice your plate is overflowing with food. Listen to what people say about the restaurants they recommend: "They really give you your money's worth. You won't go away hungry. Even Joe (the big eater) couldn't finish the prime rib. The fish fry hung over the plate." When I was coaching, the guys loved eating in places with a buffet. They were cheap and filling. I never went with them and I drove the point home, "I don't feed out of troughs."

In Summary

- Know what you are eating.
- Know how much you are eating.
- Calories matter.
- Control the size of your portions.
- Don't eat mindlessly.
- Don't eat when you are distracted.
- Don't eat while you are driving or even sitting in your car.
- Don't eat while watching TV, in a movie, or reading the newspaper.
- Eat complex carbohydrates, not simple sugars.
- Slow down.
- Do the recommended mental exercises.

7

Diet Strategies

Throughout this book, I have been discussing strategies concerning diet and weight loss. As I mentioned in the introduction this isn't meant to be a diet book, but only about why and how we gain weight. It is common knowledge that before you can change you must first become aware of the problem. The first step of Alcoholics Anonymous is facing the demon by admitting: I am an alcoholic. I think it is pretty obvious why obesity is rampant in North America. We eat too much of the wrong foods, and we've become too lazy or too overworked and stressed-out to exercise. This brings up the next Commandment: **You didn't gain the weight overnight, so don't expect to lose it overnight**.

The easiest way to understand this commandment is to reemphasize the contribution that calories make to weight gain or loss. This may get a little depressing because it will demonstrate how only a few extra calories will dramatically affect your weight over time. If you allow your child to drink 8 ounces of juice more than he needs daily, he will gain 10 pounds in a year. Conversely let's say that you are adamant about losing weight and have figured out that your BMR is 2200 calories. If you decide to cut out 100 calories per day (now eating 2100 calories) you will only lose 10 pounds in a year. While that may be an accomplishment (it sure beats gaining 10 pounds), it becomes discouraging when you consider how long it took and how strict you had to be to lose the weight. More commonly, you decide to cut out 200 calories per day (you will begin to psychologically feel this restriction). It will take 18 days to amass the deficit of 3600 calories in order to lose 1 pound of real weight. More impressively, over a year this would add up to 20 pounds. I'm sure that most of us would be happy with losing this amount of weight, but few of us are dedicated enough to do so.[1]

I have heard many people complain they can't lose weight. A few years ago 18 people at work went on a diet that I prescribed for one week. We lost a total of 100 pounds, which is over 5 pounds per person even though a few didn't lose any. Those who didn't lose assured me that they strictly followed the diet. I didn't believe them because we were eating somewhere around 1000 calories per day. In a week we would accumulate a deficit of 5000 to 15,000 calories resulting in 1 to 3 pounds weight loss in the week.[2] How is it possible not to lose weight when you are on a diet? Even more dramatically, how is possible to lose only 10 pounds in a year on some highly promoted diet? All you need to do is analyze what you eat to get the answer.

Let's assume that you go on a 1500 calorie diet and your BMR is 2200 calories. Now we are talking real dietary restriction. Your mind begins to play games with you: "I'm starving...I feel light-headed...This finger full of frosting won't count." In two weeks you will rack up a deficit of 9800 calories or 2¾ pounds.[3]

---

[1] Recall that the studies comparing the most popular diets demonstrated an average 10 pound weight loss for those who remained on them for a full year. What's the point of subscribing to some diet that's in-vogue when you could lose 20 pounds in a year by cutting 200 calories (one 16 oz beer or soda) per day?

[2] As I said before, much of the initial, rapid loss of weight can be attributed to water weight.

Not bad but not overly impressive for the amount of work that you had to do. You decide to continue the diet for another 4 weeks because you are getting married, and you want to be able to wear that dress. On your wedding day everyone tells you how good you look. You confide to your bridesmaids how hard it was to lose those 10 pounds (2.7 X 3 = 8.2 pounds + a little water weight).

It's time to party! You eat everything in sight, including a large piece of wedding cake. It's your day. You've been looking forward to the honeymoon cruise. For the next week you lie in the sun on deck sipping piña coladas. The nice thing about the cruise is that you can eat all day long, and the food is so good. When you get back home you are appalled and dismayed that you've gained back 8 pounds. Impossible! You were more active than normal: swimming and walking.

Too bad you didn't realize (or admit to yourself) that you were consuming 4000 calories per day, much of it sugary alcoholic drinks, desserts and salty, high fat foods. While you raised your BMR to 2500 through all the activity, you ate a surplus of 1500 calories daily.[4] Now you're really discouraged. While you lose some of the water weight you go back to eating 2700 calories per day because you are cooking for 2, you don't want to waste the food, and you've been going over to relatives' and friends' houses for dinner with your new husband. In one month you've gained almost all of your weight back![5]

Let me give you one more common example. Again you are on a 1500 calorie diet. In two weeks you lose almost 3 pounds. You decide to splurge on the weekend eating pizza, chicken

---

[3] 700 X 14 days = 9800 calories / 3600 calories per pound = 2.7 pounds.

[4] 1500 X 8 days = 12000 calories / 3600 = 3.3 pounds + salt-retaining water weight.

[5] 500 X 30 days = 15000 calories / 3600 = 4.2 pounds.

wings and drinking beer during the football game. Over the weekend you consume over 8400 calories. The deficit of 9800 calories is cut in half by your rewarding yourself.[6] You relax over the next 2 weeks and you are back to where you started. It doesn't take long to realize that all your efforts didn't work. You convince yourself that you can't lose weight or dieting doesn't work for you.

Dieting won't work unless you are committed for the long haul. Only when you finally come to this conclusion will you understand that you are not dieting, but you are changing the way that you eat and how you approach eating:

- No one can diet forever.
- Thin people are thin because they eat differently, not because they diet.
- Portion size and calories are important.
- You can reward yourself: only do so mindfully, and not routinely.
- Don't let the pounds slowly accumulate. It will take you a long time to get rid of them.
- Think weight maintenance.

You are what you drink

The next Commandment is one of the easiest diet strategies: **Don't drink your calories.** This is common sense. Why drink 2 cans of soda at 150 calories apiece when you can have a good size dish of pasta instead? It really doesn't matter what you are drinking: 150 calories of beer is the same as 150 calories of pop, is the same as 150 calories of juice.[7] Calories are calories.

---

[6] 8400 calories – 4400 calories (BMR X 2) = 4000 calories.
9800 – 4000 = 5800 calorie deficit.

[7] A study by the International Association for the Study of Obesity (April 2007) found that 75% of German men and 60% of women are overweight or

It amazes me that we don't recognize one of today's biggest diet problems. Everywhere you go you see people drinking from plastic tubs.

Somehow we got confused when it was recommended we drink more fluids during the day. Instead of water we've gone to soda, both sugar-filled and sugar-free. To repeat, rats given sugar substitute ate three times more than rats given sugar. I am not convinced that diet sodas are any better than regular soda when it comes to weight maintenance, and I can't believe that the chemicals in the drinks are good for you. I remember riding my bike as a kid to one of the very first fast food joints, in order to pick up some milk shakes. We were playing football in the street and a few of us went to buy drinks for the rest. When we got back the shakes had shrunk down to half their original volume. It didn't take a genius to figure that they were chock-full of enhancers and stabilizers. I'm not saying that you cannot drink anything other than water, just be mindful that we often overlook the calories in drinks.

I have heard it said that this is the food planet. We are always eating and drinking. Food is prominent in our mythology: Mother Earth feeds us and we are devoured by Father Time. What's eating you today? I can't believe what we are fed by the media!

We all recognize that feeding an animal is the best way to train it. Petting zoos are filled with little kids befriending ducks and goats and horses with an appropriate morsel of food. Food and drink are our security blanket. Perhaps this is why everyone is sipping from a cup, chewing gum or carrying around a bottle of water. I remember sending one of my rowing boats out to compete in the National Championships. I watched as they pulled away from the dock, expecting them to exude

---

obese. One researcher from University of Munich admitted, "Germans are some of the biggest beer drinkers in the world."

confidence and determination for the task ahead. When the boat stopped to allow the rowers to adjust their equipment, I was appalled to see them take water bottles up to their lips. The only image that stuck in my mind was that they were sucking on baby bottles. While we all need to drink enough water, too many of us use it as a security blanket.[8] Like all eating, there is a time and a place, and to everything there is a season.

Salt of the earth

Sodium and potassium are the most critical ions in the body. Their proper balance is required for nerve conduction, muscle contraction and heart rhythm. Yet table salt is the most common toxin contained in our diet. Sodium chloride leaches out potassium from the body. Salt can be poisonous to animals and infants and has been used in some societies as a suicidal agent. Remember those shipwreck movies, when the weakest in the lifeboat broke down and drank sea water to quench his thirst, only to hasten his death. I am sure that you've woken up with parched lips and tongue after eating salty foods like pizza and chips. Your body has been poisoned by the salt and is craving water. Interestingly, you may have experienced the same sensation after eating out in certain restaurants. Tells you something about how they're preparing their food to make it more palatable doesn't it?

People from cultures that do not add salt to food have no high blood pressure.[9] When salt is added to taste, there is a ten-fold increase in the risk of developing hypertension. If salt is added before tasting the risk increases one hundred-fold. A natural

[8] Recently a number of deaths during marathons have been attributed to hyponatremia (low blood sodium). The runners have been so indoctrinated that they are drinking themselves to death.

[9] "Without exception, low blood pressure societies are low salt societies." JAMA 237: 1305, 1397-1408, 1977. Quoted by R. Ballentine, M.D. in Diet and Nutrition, Himalayan International Institute, Honesdale, Pa., 1978.

balance of sodium and potassium is contained in fresh fruits and vegetables. The addition of table salt is an acquired, unnecessary habit. Perhaps we all need to add a little salt to maximize flavor of the foods we cook—just don't put a shaker on the table.

In Summary

- Forget about dieting. Think about eating properly.
- Weight loss and ultimately weight maintenance are long term goals.
- Be mindful of what and when you eat and drink.
- Don't drink your calories.
- Drink chemical-free bottled water.
- Once cooked, don't add salt to your food. Leave the shaker off the table.

8

Don't Bother Exercising

Eating alone will not keep a man well; he must also take exercise. For food and exercise, while possessing opposite qualities work together to produce health. It is the nature of exercise to use up material, but of food and drink to make good deficiencies...Hippocrates.

We've arrived at Commandment 9: **Walk more.** This forms the second pillar of the weight maintenance paradigm. The first pillar was to eat less. As I have already said, I prefer not to use the term exercise because of the connotation. I can only picture in my head obese people dancing or jumping around on those Richard Simmons' videos. While it is an admirable way to burn up more calories, it can't be good for their tendons and joints. Many obese people that I see can barely walk, much less do jumping jacks.

Have you ever noticed when you are on a diet you get more tired or more accurately, you don't want to do too much? It would seem to be common sense that if you take in less energy, you will have less energy to expend. However, that is not what is happening. While I admit that when I am on a restrictive diet regimen I want to do less, I have found that I actually need less sleep. It is not as if the body is more tired, but it does feel like it has slowed down. We come up against another one of our bodies' fundamental survival strategies: our metabolism slows down to prevent body wasting and ultimately starvation and death. Like the hibernating bear we tend to pack the pounds on during the winter—traditionally a time during which we had less access to food. Similar to the bear which actually sleeps during the time of less food, our metabolism dramatically slows down when we diet.

Try this experiment:

- Find out your average resting pulse rate and then compare it to your pulse rate when you have been on a diet for a while.

You will see that after dieting, your resting pulse rate goes down. Your body is conserving energy (your BMR decreases). That is why over time it becomes more difficult to lose weight. I have dealt with quite a few anorexics. They restrict their diets to such a degree that their BMR drops very low—sometimes you see heart rates in the low 40's. They intuitively recognize this and so they keep increasing their level of activity. I remember a young woman that was hospitalized for this very serious eating disorder who continuously marched through the hallways of the hospital, defeating every effort to put on needed pounds. She eventually starved herself to death. Every now and then I notice an extraordinarily thin woman jogging around the local streets and I'm sure I am seeing the same mindset.

I mention this example to reinforce the principle that whenever you diet you must increase your level of activity. Recall the healthy centenarians when they remain active, and the walking New Yorkers. Compare that with the increasing obesity in our children who are planted in front of the TV or video game, especially at a time when there has been a decrease in physical education in the schools. Increased physical activity is crucial for proper weight maintenance. I'm not minimizing the healthful effects that activity has on heart and lung function, but I am stressing that it raises your BMR.

In research based on U.S. Department of Education data, a study determined that five hours of physical education per week would produce a 43% reduction in the number of kindergarten girls who were overweight.[1]   Because a similar reduction was not found in boys, it was postulated that boys are more active at this age and they would experience a similar benefit a few years later.

Television, video games, computers and automobiles have contributed to the decrease of physical activity in our children. Years ago our suburban streets were filled with kids playing pick up games—now they are eerily silent. After getting off a plane in Rome, I drove to the hill-town of Spoleto. It was around noon and I didn't realize that Italy closed down from 12 to 3 PM to enable the people to leisurely consume their mid-day meal. Trying to fight off the jet-lag, I sat on a bench with my wife waiting for the church to open for visitors. Hearing little footsteps I turned to watch some nuns leading about 25 school children into the piazza. It was an idyllic scene—all the kids were in uniform as they skipped in line down the cobblestone entry-way. Suddenly squeals reverberated off the surrounding stone buildings as they began running all over the square, into the corners, up to the 700 year old statues and onto the foundation of the central fountain. This activity went on for more than an hour. I don't think that this was gym period, or some physical education hour precisely coordinated by some certified professional to burn off the right amount of calories. It was just kids being allowed to freely run around the piazza enjoying games of tag, or singing and dancing—in other words, playing!

---

[1] It estimated that the obesity rate of 5-6 year old girls would decrease from 10% to 5.8%.

In North America our children's physical activity is dependent upon parents.[2] We drive them to dance class, hockey, soccer practice or karate—all organized activities that are managed by adults. How often do your kids go to the park and play baseball or football with their friends in pick-up games? I remember the entire neighborhood coming over to our house in West Virginia after dinner to play capture-the-flag for a couple of hours. We want our kids to be active, yet we don't encourage them to be so on their own. For too many, physical activity has become a chore. If exercise has to be managed and controlled by adults, why do you think our kids retreat back into their rooms, or in front of the TV, hypnotizing themselves with a video game? We are conditioning our children to delineate certain periods of time for "exercise" instead of fostering an active life-style. When exercise is relegated to some specific block of time, what will happen when that time inevitably becomes more constrained?

In an article entitled, "Obesity in Britain: gluttony or sloth?" it was noted that the obesity rate increased 150% from 1980 to 1995. Because energy and fat intake actually decreased during this same period, the authors deduced that the reason for the increase was a less active population.[3] It is well-known that an active lifestyle has numerous positive effects on health including lowering blood pressure and abdominal fat, and improving the blood lipid profile and effectiveness of insulin. These beneficial effects result in a lower incidence of death from chronic diseases such as arteriosclerosis, heart disease, cancer and diabetes.

In a study from the National Heart, Lung and Blood Institute comparing lifestyle effects on blood lipid profiles, it was found that exercise significantly improved high-density lipoprotein

---

[2] Children with more active parents are more active themselves.

[3] Prentice, A.M., and S.A. Jebb. British Medical Journal 311: 437-439, 1995.

cholesterol (HDL-C), even without weight loss.[4]   Using information from MRI scans researchers in London have created "fat maps" showing where people store fat. They have found that people who maintain their weight by diet rather than exercise are likely to have major deposits of internal fat, even if they are thin. What are <u>you</u> really like on the inside?

Numerous studies have shown that while more weight is lost through diet alone when compared to exercise alone, the combination of diet and exercise was the best regimen. Not only did it produce the most weight loss, but more of the weight lost was body fat and the weight was kept off for a longer period of time.[5] It is obvious why this occurs when we analyze calories. When you run slowly for an hour (and how many of us are capable of doing so?), you burn up about 600 calories. A Big-Mac, 32-ounce soda or super-size fries <u>each</u> contain more calories than that. All that work passes out the window when you reach for your food at the drive-thru!

The athlete's experience

Like most men I enjoy watching sports. However, I prefer to watch endurance events versus games because during a marathon or a triathlon, the athlete's body and will are always on the line. Too often when I watch a football game I see big men sitting on benches or standing around with hands on hips and huge stomachs bulging out. There is too much stoppage of play, especially for commercials. I can appreciate the power and skills of the players, but I do not believe they are physiologically stressed like the long distance, individual athlete.

---

[4] Interestingly, alcohol consumption provided the largest improvement in HDL, and cigarette smoking actually lowered HDL levels. One thing I didn't mention in the review of the centenarian populations is that they all drank alcohol daily!

[5] Stanford Weight Control Project, 1991.

A few years ago I saw parts of the Tour de France. It's unfortunate that scandals of drug use and blood doping dominate the news of the race. We forget that the competitors are still riding 100-150 miles per day for almost 3 weeks. They are peddling for upwards of 8 hours daily and burning up as much as 9,000 calories. What do they eat? They ride along picking high-energy bars, bread, fruit, water and power drinks out of cloth sacks that are handed to them by their support crews. They are not forcing down a huge burger and fries, or sucking on a Big-Gulp. While the athletes know that they need high energy foods, I find it telling that they don't eat a donut or potato chips on the road. They concentrate on easily digested, readily absorbed foods that allow them to sustain extreme physical exertion. You won't find an Atkins aficionado among them.

In the late 1970's the Ironman Triathlon in Hawaii caught the imagination of the public. In 1982, 50% of the competitors followed the same low fat, high carbohydrate regimen of multi-race winner Dave Scott. He was a strict adherent to the Pritikin diet.[6] His diet was composed of 10% fat, 15% protein and 75% complex carbohydrate. As I've mentioned, the body uses mainly carbohydrate for fuel. All the long distance athletes understand this and they manipulate their diets accordingly.

The athlete's experience is that they need complex carbohydrates to maintain their energy. Even if you are not an athlete you should take note. Not only does the athlete's diet provide energy to race and train 6-8 hours per day, but it is also the best diet for health. Pritikin originally developed his diet to lower fats and cholesterol in the blood, and halt—if not reverse—the effects of arteriosclerosis. Unfortunately as the long-term study of diets has shown, the more extreme are the

---

[6] Nathan Pritikin was the founder and director of the Pritikin Longevity Centers in California and Pennsylvania. He wrote numerous books on health and diet including The Pritikin Promise, and The Pritikin Program for Diet and Exercise.

hardest to follow, and have the highest drop-out rates. While I realize that it's very difficult to limit the daily dietary fat to 10%, it is important to recognize that a diet high in complex carbohydrates and low in fat is ultimately the healthiest one. Any diet that substitutes high fat foods for complex carbohydrates goes against most medical recommendations, athletic experience and common sense.

I am not advocating strictly following the Pritikin diet, although it would be beneficial for those who have serious cardiovascular disease. If your arteries are lined with fat—cut way back on dietary fat. People are stubborn however. Many with chronic lung disease caused by smoking won't even give up cigarettes! One of the concerns about a high carbohydrate, low fat and low protein diet would be not getting enough protein. Staying with the athlete experience: what about the pre-fight or pre-game routine of the large steak? It is obvious that the muscles of the endurance athlete function well, even without a lot of protein in the diet. You must <u>understand that a diet high in complex carbohydrates actually decreases the need for protein: in effect, it is "protein sparing"</u>. How much protein do you need? Massively muscled gorillas are strict vegetarians.

The major reason for the increase in height noted by the National Center for Health Statistics is improved nutrition.[7] The average soldier in WWII was 5'5", now he is 5'9½". The Japanese have shown even more remarkable gains in height. These improvements are not all attributed to protein intake. Improved nutrition means a more balanced and readily available food supply. The USDA recommends that protein should contribute 12% of the daily calories (note that in the Pritikin diet, protein supplies 15%).

Most of us believe that only meat, fish, poultry and dairy products contain protein. In 1910, meat, fish and poultry

---

[7] The average height of both men and women has increased by 1 inch from 1960-62 to 1999-2001.

supplied 30% of the total daily calories from protein with dairy supplying 16% and plant sources providing the remaining 54%. Today we get 70% of our protein from animal and dairy products, even though nutritionists believe that the healthy, balanced diet should derive only 33% from animal sources and 67% from plants.

We all eat more than enough protein!   An interesting explanation for the persistent belief in the strength-giving properties of meat is that meat adds aggression, not just protein. Compare the mindset of the endurance athlete to that of the boxer or the football player. In India, most Hindus are vegetarian while the Sikhs eat meat.   Perhaps it is not a coincidence that the Sikhs traditionally have made up the police force and the military.

How much exercise is enough?

In the early 1970's Dr. Kenneth Cooper founded the Cooper Institute for Aerobics Research in Dallas, Texas. The Institute began a long-term study on the effects of physical fitness on survival.   It found that in men physical fitness ranked just behind avoidance of high cholesterol and having neither parent die from coronary artery disease. In women, being physically fit was the most important determinant of long-term survival.[8]

Today, most of us are familiar with the term aerobic, referring to the type of activity that was shown to benefit heart and lung function. It is recommended that you get 20-30 minutes of aerobic activity three times per week in order to insure cardiovascular fitness.   Aerobic activity is that which is performed with a heart rate of 100 to 120 beats per minute.[9]

---

[8] The Aerobics Center Longitudinal Study, 1989.

[9] There are many different formulas in use in order to calculate your heart-rate zone, but it is probably sufficient to assume 100-120 beats per minute.

As the title of this chapter suggests, forget about exercising. Walking at a brisk pace will probably raise your heart rate to these levels. I'm not recommending that you have to march through the streets swinging your arms wildly. Swinging your arms back and forth across your chest only serves to put more stress on your trunk. It's not a very efficient way to maintain forward momentum. <u>Walk like you enjoy it, not like you are ready to punch someone</u>!

While it is admirable to exercise strenuously for 90 minutes along with a famous instructor on video-tape, it doesn't take long before it becomes a chore, or you get injured. In one study, over 50% of aerobics instructors had suffered an injury in the 6 months prior to the survey. Those were <u>instructors</u>, not overweight, out-of-shape students. Consulting energy expenditure tables (for a 175 pound person):

- Aerobics, 804 calories per hour.
- Running 8 minutes per mile, 990 calories.
- Bicycle racing, 810 calories per hour.
- Lawn mowing, 540 calories per hour.
- Brisk walking, 486 calories.
- Bicycling leisurely at 9 mph, 480 calories.

Note that the only two "exercises" that could be sustained by most people are leisurely biking and brisk walking and both activities burn up almost 500 calories per hour. Adding 1 hour of walking to your normal routine would enable you to calculate your daily caloric need as BMR X 1.5 (the multiplier for moderate activity). If you increase walking to 2 hours daily, you would increase your BMR X 1.7 (very active).[10]

I can hear it now: How can I walk 2 hours per day? If I had that much time I could go to the gym, or I wouldn't be so negligent about my health. However, adding an evening walk may

_____

[10] See Chapter 6, page 54.

actually be enjoyable, and help you digest your meal. Studies have shown that lying down (watching TV?) after eating increases the chances of obesity and gastro-esophageal reflux disease. Walking an hour in the evening can become part of your routine.

In order to add the other hour you have to change how you do things during the day:

- Walk to and from the bus stop with your children.
- Park in the back of the parking lot.
- Use the stairs at work.
- Walk during your lunch hour.
- Walk to a fellow employee's work-space instead of sending an email.
- Use a push mower instead of a riding mower.
- Rake the leaves instead of using one of those noise-polluting blowers.
- Walk your dog instead of letting him out in the backyard to bark annoyingly at your neighbors.
- Take advantage of the local bicycle lanes and nature walks.
- Ask yourself throughout the day: is what I am doing helping me to increase my level of activity? If not—find another way.

9

Change Your Mindset

In a society that assures us that more is better, it is not always easy to trust that we have enough, that we are enough. We have to cut through the illusion that abundance is security, and trust that we don't have to buffer ourselves against reality. We have learned to trust abundance, we can learn to trust simplicity. We can practice simplicity.[1]

All the information that I have presented up to now leads us to the last Commandment: **To change your set point you must change your mindset**.

It should be pretty obvious that we have been off course for many years now. We've gotten heavier by eating more and becoming more sedentary. We have allowed the food industry to dictate our tastes so that we no longer even know what good, nutritious food is. Convenience is a killer! We've gotten away from simple, natural, real foods. We are gullible

---

[1] John Daido Loori, The Zen of Creativity, p.166. Ballantine Books, New York, NY, 2004.

enough to believe that any new diet will work, without ever changing our eating patterns or lifestyle. Worst of all, we're passing all these habits on to our children.

This book has been written to heighten your awareness to the relationship we all have with food. Similar to other relationships, this one can also be dysfunctional. I don't write these words in an attempt to deliver more pop psychology. There already is enough self-analysis and self-concern in the world today.[2] However, it is important to realize that each one of us thinks about food and eating in a unique way. I adopted two feral kittens who were living in my neighbor's abandoned chicken coop. They matured into beautiful, long-haired cats: one is white and the other calico. From the beginning the calico cat ate much more food and subsequently became quite fat. She stares at her sister while she eats, waiting to pounce on any uneaten morsels of food. If my wife gives the white cat an extra treat, the calico sulks and wears an expression of disappointment. The calico cat has the mindset of a fat person.

I'm sorry if this sounds harsh, but I'm trying to shake you from your comfort zone. I'm amazed that almost every time I ask a patient with abdominal pain what she ate the night before, trying to find out whether a high fat meal was consumed causing a gall bladder problem, she answers, "Some salad…crackers…and…a bowl of cereal." I recently saw a young woman suffering from an attack who admitted she ate 2 fillet-of-fish sandwiches and a large fry at McDonald's. She turned to her husband and said, "Then we ate a big tub of popcorn dripping in butter at the show." At first I was stunned. I looked at the woman and we both

---

[2] Narcissism: the excessive interest in oneself and one's physical appearance.

started laughing. I patted her on the back and said, "At last...an honest patient!"

I am sure that you've known an obese person whom you never saw eat. Have you heard the term "closet eater"? How many times have you popped something into your mouth thinking that if no one else knows—or you swallow it fast enough—it doesn't count? These are all tricks we perform so we can say: "I don't know why I can't lose weight!" If you can't be honest with yourself you will never be able to solve the problem.

The first step in Alcoholics Anonymous is to admit that you are an alcoholic. I have the mindset of a fat person. I think about food all the time. I worry about what I'm having for dinner, or if my wife is making enough. I am a master at planning trips even in foreign countries. I read guidebooks and study maps that enable me to eat in the right restaurant at the right time with the least amount of extra effort. For example, if I'm going to the Museum of Natural History in New York City, I get there by 9:00 AM which allows me to view the exhibit for 2-3 hours and walk to a nice restaurant on the upper west side for lunch. There are three reasons why I am not obese (while still being overweight): first, I walk a lot, and work out strenuously for 20-30 minutes 3 days a week; second, I practice much of what I preach (e.g. don't drink your calories); lastly, my wife does not have the mindset of a fat person. I live with a person who will not eat if she's not hungry (hard to believe). She leaves food on her plate when she is satiated (God forbid). She doesn't question at every restaurant whether we've ordered enough (aghast). Finally, she regulates her eating by how her clothes feel (not me, I just suck my gut in a little more).

Psychology of food

There are many reasons why we all have a unique relationship with food. Sigmund Freud labeled the first stage of psychological development the oral stage. After a short period of complete attachment to the mother the infant begins to explore her world with her hands. When she starts to crawl around she tries to digest her explorations by placing everything into her mouth. Every parent recognizes this stage and tries to keep the infant safe by guiding and correcting her behavior. If this is done with enough love and understanding, while the child will always have some residual dissatisfaction with the parent, she will develop normally.[3]   The implications of this process cannot be overstated.   If there is conflict in the home, too stern correction of the child's behavior, or ignorance of the child's needs the child may become fixated (Freud's term) at this stage.[4]

We have all experienced the comfort that food provides. Obviously it is satisfying our need for sustenance, but sustenance is both physical and emotional. Even with a fairly healthy relationship with food we are all still capable of regressing to the oral stage of development at times of stress. "Food makes me happy...I need a piece of chocolate...a cup of coffee...a drink!" I stated in the very beginning—that's okay. We are all human beings with the same needs and desires and weaknesses. What makes us different and unique is how we individually manage those traits. Know thyself! Be honest with yourself. Open your eyes. Wake up. Change your mindset.

---

[3] There will always be some conflict or complex because the parent is restricting what the child is demanding—a clash of wills.

[4] Needs are both for love and guidance: "if one is fed sweets all the time she becomes sick."

In his book, Daido Loori continues, "To be simple means to make a choice about what's important, and to let go of all the rest."[5] What's important to you? Because you are reading this book I have to assume that weight loss and maintenance are important. You still must ask yourself why you want to lose weight, and is it important enough to you? How committed are you? We've been conditioned throughout our lives to use food as a security blanket. It's time to recognize that food provides only a false shelter. Strip away the veneer of emotional satisfaction and societal conformity and step out into the light. Your first steps may be hesitant, and you may even retreat back under cover, but over time, with enough effort, you may actually change the way you view food and eating, and your attachment to them. Only then will you change your mindset.

Food as ritual

Throughout our lives we swing on a pendulum between the states of expansion and constriction: "I want to consume everything around me...I must deny myself any pleasure." We are in search of balance. We all know the jovial, fat person stereotype—happy, laughing, enthusiastically consuming life. Compare that to the miserly, old man—hyper-disciplined, rigid, unwilling or unable to express and experience joy. Either state in the extreme is unhealthy. One must strive for balance and "let go of all the rest." Be content.

Contentment is an invisible spiritual force. Like spice in food, it is the secret ingredient that makes life rich and satisfying. Contentment affirms life, it does not restrict it. Learn to moderate your ambition. If you are constantly

---

[5] The Zen of Creativity, p.154.

seeking that which cannot reasonably be obtained you will never know happiness—you will never be content. The recognition of your own abilities naturally leads to contentment and with it comes security. Our inability to do so forces us to search outside of ourselves for fulfillment, and this may help to explain the underlying disillusionment that we feel about modern life. Technology has quickened the pace of life and makes us believe that we can solve any problem and obtain anything we want.[6] However, we all come to realize that this is not true and ultimately we have to face the fact that security is not "out there". Only when you accept that security is an inner experience will you no longer need to hide behind food (or someone or thing other than yourself like your parents, husband, job, government or religion). Remember that all religious creeds are trying to release you from your chains. <u>In the end however, it is your responsibility to step away from the chains that have been cut away</u>.

Recently I saw a very disturbing image on TV when a small child, who had been held as one of the captives by the terrorists in Beslan, Russia, was blown out of the school gym by a detonated bomb. The photographer who witnessed the event related his horror as he snapped a picture of the child climbing back through the window and back to her captors. While she was eventually freed, all she had to do is walk away from the gym but instead went back inside—back to captivity.

Perhaps you think that I must have gotten side-tracked. I was talking about food and now I mention religion.[7]

---

[6] Anyone can grow up to be President or drive the car of his dreams (just lease it).

[7] It's not such a stretch. Alcoholics Anonymous is loaded with religious connotations.

Unfortunately I believe that one of the fundamental defects of modern life is that we have moved too far away from the sacred. We've tried to sever the connection through our intelligence and reason. I had the privilege to see 12,000 year old etchings of deer, bear and buffalo drawn on cave walls in the Vézère Valley in France. Primitive people had made these elaborate, yet tender drawings of animals that they were hunting. What was most interesting is that the hunters did not live in the dark, mysterious confines of the caves, for they were often inhabited by dangerous animals. Instead, the caves were considered places of worship, and the artists were paying homage to the animals that they ate. The caves were temples and their food was sacred. What's even more eerie is that both my wife and I thought the cave smelled like incense—perhaps from the moss on the walls— perhaps not!

Traditionally man has used ritual to elevate his state of consciousness—to rise above the mundane world—to worship. Most religions include eating of the sacred food, whether it is manna from heaven, bread and wine, the Last Supper or the church social. <u>Aided by ritual and ceremony, food is made sacred by sitting at the Table</u>.

The symbolism of the meal is personally meaningful because it outwardly embodies an inner process. An earlier chapter advised that food should be your medicine, and now I am taking it one step further: food should be sacred. We are fed by the ceremony and presentation of the meal as much as we are fed by the food itself. Be mindful of the food you eat because it nourishes your soul as much as your body. Elevate the experience of eating above consumption, to appreciation of the gift that has been given to you. Just because you don't need to kill the sacrificial lamb doesn't mean that you would no longer benefit from the ritual of the meal. Perhaps the real values of a prayer before eating include:

- Reinforcing the ritual of the meal.
- Slowing down the pace of daily life and preparing your body.
- Making you more aware of the moment and the task at hand.

In his "Verses for Eating Mindfully" Thich Nhat Hanh prays:

> In this food,
> I see clearly the presence
> Of the entire universe
> Supporting my existence.

Be vigilant

When I talk about mindset I mean all the things that take place inside your head. These include the thoughts and the games that you play with yourself so that you can rationalize why and what you're eating. Realize that your desires can sneak up and ambush you. I have told myself that I'll have self-control at work and then I eat 4 slices of pizza. Afterwards I'm disgusted and I think: "From this day forward I won't let it happen again." The next day somebody buys donuts...

Go slow

One of the real problems that we have concerning our weight is that we are searching for the miracle cure.[8] We all expect to latch on to some external program that will change

---

[8] See Chapter 7. **You didn't gain the weight overnight, so don't expect to lose it overnight.**

our internal relationship to food. It can't happen that way. You must give up the idea that there is a rapid or short-term solution. It is important to realize that weight maintenance is a lifelong process—one that will never be over.   It is necessary to start slowly but be steadfast. In that way you will become more sensitive to all the factors that influence how you approach food and diet.   You will begin to understand that you are living on the food planet, and much of what you experience in life revolves around nourishment, satiation and fulfillment. The relationship that you have with your world becomes more fathomable and therefore more enjoyable. <u>You are part of life—not apart from life</u>.[9]

In Conclusion

- It is your relationship to food that determines your weight.
- Be honest with yourself.
- Stand in front of the mirror (preferably undressed) and look at yourself.
- Judge your weight by how your clothes feel—if they're too tight, cut back.
- Emotional security comes from within you—not from outside you. Not from food.
- Do you need to eat or drink something as an emotional pick-me-up? Try to be aware of those times. Better yet, recognize what situations force you into those needs, and avoid them.
- Food should be sacred.
- The meal should be a ritual—a ceremony.[10]

---

[9] Goswami Kriyananda, personal communication.

[10] Don't let your husband wear a dirty white tee-shirt at the dinner table. He wouldn't go to church like that.

- Don't let your guard down!
- Don't expect miracles—make weight maintenance part of your life.

10

Set Point

It should be obvious by now that proper weight maintenance is vital to living an active healthy life. Unfortunately it's always easier to put on weight than it is to take it off. It also seems that after losing weight, it comes right back on leaving us back where we started, if not heavier. It is almost as if we have a set point for weight that is difficult to change. Perhaps it's all about survival: the body always wants to maintain a positive energy state to protect itself against starvation. Throughout human history those who survived were the ones who were best able to live off the fat of the land. Too bad in today's time of plenty, we've become the fat land.

Building blocks

It is important that our bodies function properly. Structure and function are actually the products of protein metabolism because muscles, tendons, ligaments, hormones, enzymes and much of the body's cellular structure are protein based. Weight maintenance therefore can be thought of as providing the body's protein requirement. Carbohydrates are the primary source of energy and for the brain, they are the only source. I am sure you have noticed how you get light-headed when your blood sugar level drops. With the use of insulin,[1] the sugar level can become dangerously low leading to disorientation, coma and death. Fat is the storage form of energy. <u>Once you consume more calories than you burn off, those calories, whether they come from fat, carbohydrate or protein, are stored as fat</u>.

Proteins are chains of amino acids but these chains cannot be absorbed intact.[2] After the protein is broken down through digestion, the amino acids are absorbed individually. The liver filters out the amino acids and they are reconstituted into labile protein, sent and incorporated into muscle, connective tissue and nervous system protein or if in excess, converted into carbohydrate and stored as fat. In this case, the amine portion of the amino acid is broken off and excreted in the urine as ammonia. High levels of ammonia are toxic in the blood stream. In fact, the ammonia level is the most important measurement of liver failure. This helps to explain the toxicity and bad breath associated with high protein (e.g. low carbohydrate) diets. Besides, protein is the least efficient source of energy, and by far the most expensive. Like all protein, meat must be broken down into its constituent amino acids. However, analysis has shown that only about 50% of the protein in meat is absorbed. In contrast, almost 90% of the protein in egg is absorbed.

Labile protein comprises 5% of the total protein pool and it is the portion most responsive to dietary protein. A low protein

---

[1] The major function of insulin is to facilitate the entry of glucose into the cells.

[2] Any supplement that is a large protein molecule (e.g. an animal hormone) must be broken down first. It will no longer be the molecule it once was, or it was sold as. <u>Don't be misled. Dietary supplements of enzymes and hormones cannot be absorbed intact by the body</u>.

diet will deplete the labile pool in 3-5 days. After this period, loss of protein from the body progresses at a slower, steady state. It takes over 20 days on a protein deficient diet before the much larger muscle and connective tissue protein pools even start to be consumed. The last storage pool of protein, the nervous system, begins to be affected at 90 days.

It has been said that protein is memory. If the nervous system is mainly protein, and protein is responsible for most structure and function, then the body's set point is protein dependent. **To change the set point requires a change in protein storage and metabolism**. Most diets ignore this principle. Could this be the reason all diets fail? Simply stated, decreasing the body's protein (storage) should decrease the body's size. Manipulating protein metabolism accomplishes this. A short term protein deficient diet will exhaust the labile protein pool, and force the body to convert carbohydrate and fat back into protein. Change your body's memory by changing your body's protein!

Carbohydrates, which are both sugars and starches, are absorbed as simple sugars and in larger chains. The simple sugars are used rapidly for energy[3] or converted along with the larger chains into glycogen by the liver. Glycogen is the main storage form of sugar and it is contained in the muscles (67%) and liver (29%). The glycogen stores are exhausted after 2 to 3½ hours of moderate exercise,[4] or after 3 days on a low carbohydrate diet. Once depleted, most of the energy needed by the body is supplied by the breakdown of the fat stores.

---

[3] The sugar "rush" or "high".

[4] "Hitting the wall" in a marathon.

Fat is absorbed as fatty acids and transported in the bloodstream as free fatty acids or attached to cholesterol.[5] Some fat is used to maintain cell wall structure and some is converted to steroids, but most is stored as fat or even worse, gets deposited on the walls of the blood vessels (atherosclerotic cardiovascular disease).   The amount of energy available from fat is almost limitless.   However, the intensity of exercise must be at a much lower level than if the energy was supplied by carbohydrate.   Interestingly, caffeine will stimulate the release of fatty acids from the fat stores and has a glycogen-sparing effect.

Understanding that protein is necessary for structure and carbohydrate is the main energy source, it would make sense that weight gain and loss is a function of the amount of protein and calories that you eat. How much daily protein is required?   The most recent information advises that the average adult should eat 48 grams of protein per day.[6] Biochemists have estimated that the requirement is closer to 30 grams if you analyze the actual turnover of protein that occurs daily.   Therefore, for a diet to be deficient in protein it would need to supply less than 40-50 grams of usable protein.[7]

As mentioned, if you stay on a low protein diet for 7 days, the labile protein pool is exhausted, but the protein in the structural components of the body (i.e. muscles, tendons etc.) is not yet affected. The body is forced to synthesize

---

[5] LDL and HDL cholesterol.

[6] 0.32 grams/pound X 150 pounds = 48 grams.

[7] A Whopper contains 35 grams of protein, only 17.5 grams are absorbed. Two eggs would provide 12 grams of which 10.8 grams are usable.

protein from carbohydrate. If the diet is also low in calories, the glycogen stores will be depleted as well. The carbohydrates necessary for protein synthesis and for energy must then be obtained by mobilizing the fat stores.

Will-power

We now come to the meat of the issue. Using the above information, it is reasonable to assume that the best way to change your set point is to deplete the labile protein and glycogen stores. This forces the mobilization of the fat stores.

Most experts say that a very low calorie diet doesn't work, but they aren't addressing protein. A low calorie diet will ultimately fail because it is impossible to maintain. An analysis of 1,522 weight loss programs containing 15,775 subjects demonstrated that a very low calorie diet produced the most weight loss at six months.[8] However after that period, all the studies showed a leveling off of weight loss and most subjects began to gain weight, especially the very low calorie group. **All diets work. All diets are meant to fail.**

We have all gone on a diet and after being discouraged by the initial results, especially in relation to how hard we are trying, we immediately begin to cheat. Admit it. When you don't lose weight you are not being honest with yourself as to what you are eating. Unfortunately this is where "will-power" comes in to play. Instead of berating yourself because you don't have enough will-power, realize that only when what you are trying to do is important enough to you

---

[8] Evidence-Informed Protocol for Weight Management. Minneapolis: HealthPartners Center for Health Promotion, 2004.

will the power be there. <u>Only when you are able to think the thought, will you have the will to succeed</u>.

Looking at it another way, we all have plenty of will-power for short periods of time. Recall the example of a newlywed— most brides can lose enough weight to squeeze into their wedding dresses. It's fairly easy for most pregnant women to stop drinking alcohol. I know many men who have quit smoking after their open-heart surgery. Too bad these major life-style changes are often not maintained, or had to be adopted after such a serious illness. When the thought finally becomes prominent enough we all have plenty of will-power.

Healthy weight management will only become important if it is considered something worthwhile to fight for. It should be obvious by now that you are actually fighting for your life and the quality of life. I taught a yoga class for older people and I distributed a survey asking them to tell me one thing that they would have done differently in their lives if they had the chance. The most common answer was: "I would have taken better care of my body." The most common reasons why people visit a doctor are back pain and upper respiratory infections. Both of these problems can be traced to lifestyle issues especially nutrition, obesity, activity and stress levels. A recent study from Loma Linda University demonstrated that a vegetarian diet will decrease mortality from all causes by 9% per year and from cardiovascular disease by 25%. Diet affects the quantity and quality of life.

"Human beings dare to do only those things that, in their interpretation of the world, are valuable to them."[9]

---

[9] Alfred Adler, <u>Understanding Human Nature</u>, p.87. Hazelden Foundation, Center City, Minnesota, 1998. First published in English in 1927.

Answer the following questions and consider:

- What is important to you?
- Are you interested enough in your health to pay attention to it?
- When you have enough interest in health, the ability to read your body's internal cues will naturally follow.
- The will-power to lose weight only exists when you pay attention to your diet.

The mind is like a wild horse. When it is first harnessed, it will kick and gyrate, trying to break loose again. Eventually with enough effort and gentle persuasion the horse can be trained and be ridden for work or for pleasure. Once a thought is present in your head, consider how easy it is to hold onto. I'm sure that you've been kept awake by your mind ruminating over something that needed to be done. "I can't take my mind off it...the thought keeps going through my head." Yet for some reason when you should remember something, especially when it's something that you shouldn't eat, the thought never comes up. What force could be so strong that it causes you to black out? Desires or cravings, can defeat your will-power—but only if you let them. Are they what you want or what you need?

It is possible to strengthen will-power. It can be trained, but remember, you are the only one who can train it—no one else can train your mind. The poet Rumi wrote:

> When you have eaten too much honey,
> It causes <u>you</u> a fever, not someone else;
> Your day's wages aren't given to someone else at day's end.[10]

---

[10] Camille Helminski, <u>Rumi: Jewels of Remembrance</u>, p. 135. Threshold Books, Putney, Vermont, 1996.

It's up to you. The first step has already been mentioned: pay attention to it. The second step is to discipline the body through the first step: be mindful of it. Learn to read the body's internal cues by asking:

- How does it feel now? Bored? Tired? Anxious? Depressed? Heavy?
- What would make it feel better?
- Is it hungry or full? Desiring or satisfied?

Only after you have become aware of your mind and body can you train or strengthen them. As you practice you will begin to recognize that <u>you are not your body or your mind</u>, and therefore, you have to treat them as entities separate from your self.

Try the following exercise,[11] sitting quietly, affirm:

- I have a body, but I am not my body. My body is a precious instrument that I use for experience and action in the outer world, but it is only an *instrument.*
- I have emotions, but I am not my emotions. These emotions are countless, changing and even contradictory. Because I can observe, analyze and understand them, I can learn to control, direct and utilize them.
- I have desires, but I am not my desires. They are aroused by inner physical and emotional drives yet they are influenced by things outside of me. Desires like emotions are changeable and contradictory, alternating between what is helpful to me and what is harmful.

---

[11] Roberto Assagioli, M.D., <u>Psychosynthesis</u>, p. 104. The Synthesis Center, Amherst, Mass., 2000. Originally published in 1965.

- I have thoughts, but I am not my thoughts. They flash across my mind; yet in an instant they change, subside and disappear. I must learn to guide and use my thoughts, not allowing them to control me.
- I am my will. Therefore, I choose what sensations, emotions, desires and thoughts I shall react to.

In Conclusion

- Your body has a "natural" weight—a set point.
- Protein is used for structure and function.
- The set point is your body's need for protein.
- To change the set point requires manipulation of the protein stores.
- Carbohydrates are the body's energy source.
- Fat is the energy storage vehicle.
- Weight management is mainly protein <u>and</u> calorie control.
- You have will-power for that which is important to you.
- The strength of your will becomes evident when you realize that it lies even deeper inside than sensations, emotions, desires and thoughts.
- Think the thought: **<u>think thin</u>**.

11

The Method

It's time to get to work. One last time, **Set Point** is not a diet book. I have tried to present a few principles that are meant to awaken your interest in taking charge of your life and in learning how to maintain your weight. Whatever diet program you choose to follow, try to incorporate those principles, specifically the Ten Commandments.

I read a New York Times article[1] in which the author tried to follow the recently published dietary guidelines from the USDA.[2] He wrote, "So I assumed that the new guidelines would not require any wrenching changes: A small adjustment here and there, but nothing I couldn't live with. I was wrong." An analysis of what he ate violated quite a few of the principles that I've laid out. He drank his calories; he ate processed, prepared foods; he ate dinner out and he had dessert. On a day in which he ate 3,528 calories, 480

---

[1] "Four Days on the Uncle Sam Diet," by William Grimes. The New York Times, Sunday,   January 23, 2005.

[2]www.usda.gov/wps/portal/!ut/pl_s.7_0_A/7_0_1RD?printable=true&cont entidonly=true&contendid=2005/01/0012.xml

calories were from fruit drinks (that he mistakenly labeled "fruit intake"), 400 calories from high-fat, processed granola and 500 calories from a piece of cherry pie. 1,380 wasted calories! By eating out he consumed 1,475 calories even without a drink. I agree with some of the conclusions of the article: "In the real world, of course, people regard food and its flavors as a source of pleasure…The new guidelines are not just health policy, they're cultural policy too. To comply fully, Americans will have to rethink their inherited notions of what makes a meal, and what makes a meal satisfying." However, when you honestly look at what he was eating it's easy to see why people can't lose weight.

Once again, I have to ask, what is important to you? If you want to control your weight there are some fundamental changes that you must make. What follows is a suggested method to reset your set point at a lower level. You must choose whatever method makes sense to you, but realize that any method requires some sacrifice or else you would never have any difficulty in losing weight.

Getting started

1. **Prime the fat-burning pump.** Follow a low calorie, low protein diet for at least 7 days to exhaust your labile protein and glycogen stores.

2. **Melt the fat stores.** After a week, increase the amount of calories that you consume but stay at least 500 calories below your daily requirement for two to three more weeks.

3. **Cut the salt, not your water intake.** If you eat the recommended foods your daily salt intake will drop to

as low as 500 mg.[3] You will begin to safely and naturally excrete excess water weight because you no longer need the fluid to dilute the salt. Increase the amount of water that you drink to help the body rid itself of toxins and to mobilize the fat. Fat stores have no water associated with them. Therefore, you need to provide extra water to efficiently use fat for energy.

4. **Get moving.** Increase your physical activity by at least 250 calories daily (preferably 500 calories).[4] Not only is the increased activity good for your health, but you need to compensate for the body's attempt to preserve itself by slowing its metabolism (as it tries to maintain its set point).

5. **Expectations.** You can expect to lose 5-10 pounds the first week. As has been explained, you could lose about 2-3 pounds of "real weight" and 3-7 pounds of water weight.[5] The water weight loss may be even greater due to the low sodium intake on **The Method**. At the end of three weeks you can lose 10-15 pounds total. What is even more important than the weight loss is that if you have been strict, you will also have reset your set point at a lower level.

6. **Make it last.** If you keep the Ten Commandments your new set point can be maintained indefinitely. After 6 months, if you have been lax, you can reset it again over 3 weeks. It is not unreasonable to follow **The Method** once or twice a year.

---

[3] The USDA recommends less than 2,400 mg. per day and a low salt diet in most hospitals is less than 2000 mg.

[4] Walking briskly for 30 to 60 minutes.

[5] **Calories are important**, p. 48.

7. **For more serious weight problems.**   Try **The Method** once a month—on three weeks, off one week (always following the Commandments)—until you reach your goal.

8. **Advantages:**
   - You eat readily available, easy to prepare and inexpensive foods.[6]
   - **The Method** is good for your health. It is a low salt, low fat and high fiber diet along with increased physical activity.
   - You begin to understand which foods are good for you and which are bad.
   - You reset your set point.

9. **Disadvantages:**
   - It takes real motivation to do. It is not easy.
   - It is best to do with a like-minded group of people. You need support—at least at first.
   - Other people will think you're nuts.
   - There's not much meat.
   - You begin to fixate on food (though that occurs with any diet).
   - You can't eat out, especially during the first week.
   - You have to plan the weeks so they do not coincide with other obligations, e.g. parties.[7]

---

[6] One of the attractions of programs like Jenny Craig and Weight Watchers is that they have meal plans to follow and even meals to eat. These can cost up to $400 per month. The cost may be worth it but you can do it much cheaper!

[7] I believe that it's better to avoid them altogether than to insult the hostess. I am sure you've been to a dinner party and been embarrassed when some Atkins adherent cried: "I'll just have cheese as my appetizer and meat for my main course please."

Day	Breakfast	Lunch	Dinner	Totals	
1	Bowl cereal skim milk small juice	Yogurt with 2 tbsp bran	Spinach macaroni	**Calories** Total fat Sat fat Carbs Protein Sodium Fiber	**1058** 31.1 14.8 178. 55.4 1280 14.1
2	2 hard/soft eggs 1 slice buttered toast	Apple 2 tbsp peanut butter	Green salad	**Calories** Total fat Sat fat Carbs Protein Sodium Fiber	**779** 59 17.2 43.8 25 479 9
3	Cottage cheese and peaches	Yogurt with bran	Tuna noodle	**Calories** Total fat Sat fat Carbs Protein Sodium Fiber	**1003** 24.7 10 120.8 77.5 1513 10.6
4	Bowl cereal skim milk	Peanut butter and jelly on 2 slices whole wheat	Green salad	**Calories** Total fat Sat fat Carbs Protein Sodium Fiber	**777** 35.2 7.7 100 25 510 13.2
5	Bowl of oatmeal with maple syrup	Yogurt with bran	Baked potato with spinach and/or broccoli	**Calories** Total fat Sat fat Carbs Protein Sodium Fiber	**1012** 28.7 15.9 155.3 40 495 17.1
6	2 eggs 1 slice buttered toast small juice	Fresh fruit	Green salad soup	**Calories** Total fat Sat fat Carbs Protein Sodium Fiber	**1066** 53.7 18.6 128.7 28.6 1242 23.7
7	Bowl cereal skim milk	Apple 2 tbsp peanut butter	Grill or broil chicken breast or fish, peas and carrots	**Calories** Total fat Sat fat Carbs Protein Sodium Fiber	**916** 24.2 7.8 100 81 1155 18

Staples

There are a few staples that are used repeatedly in **The Method**. Eating cereal with skim or low fat milk is nutritious and low calorie. Remember those commercials about the use of Special K in a diet? John Harvey Kellogg was the medical director of a health sanitarium in Battle Creek, Michigan. His center nursed patients back to health with a diet of high-fiber, whole grain cereals, fresh fruits and vegetables. The old-fashioned cereals are the best for the diet—shredded wheat, Grape-Nuts, All-Bran, Chex—all are low in fat. Be careful about eating corn flakes: corn is very high in simple sugars. I would also avoid granola as it tends to be high in fat and calories. Read the labels! When you eat oatmeal you can add sugar or honey, if you don't like maple syrup. I prefer the taste and the quality of pure maple syrup, over high fructose, artificially flavored pancake syrup that most people use.

Yogurt is actually just milk fermented with a bacterial culture. The main organism in yogurt is *Lactobacillus bulgaricus*, a close relative of one of the predominant colonists of your colon—*L. acidophilus.* It is known to be settling to the digestive tract, and has been used to cure both diarrhea and constipation. Adding bran to the yogurt helps in this effect. The bran can be wheat or oat, and can be found in powdered form in most health food stores. You could add All-Bran or Grape-Nuts as an alternative. Be careful about the yogurt that you choose. Low-fat, artificially sweetened yogurts have about 90 calories per 8 oz. serving, while whole-milk yogurt with fruit flavoring has about 250 calories. I usually eat plain, low-fat yogurt that I flavor with some pure maple syrup or fruit preserves. The calorie total then rises to about 180-200, but I know exactly what I'm eating.

It is easy to **make your own yogurt** with the following recipe and you don't need a yogurt maker:

- 3 cups of milk (skim, low-fat or whole)
- ½ cup plain yogurt
- Heat the milk on the stove to a boil, remove from heat and cool to lukewarm. Test with a clean spoon, not your finger.
- Add the yogurt. Cover the mixture in a bowl and ferment in a warm place overnight. I usually just place it in my shut off oven.
- You can add a packet of gelatin to the heated milk mixture if you want the yogurt to be firmer.

You should not eat commercially grown iceberg lettuce. Buy specialty salad greens because they are much higher in taste, nutritive value and freshness. Follow the old adage: "When you're green—you're clean." It is better to make your own salad dressing (i.e. fresher, lower in calories and without added preservatives, salt and sugars). **My favorite dressing** is (serves 2):

- 3 tablespoons extra virgin olive oil
- 1 teaspoon high quality balsamic vinegar
- 1 teaspoon Dijon or whole-grain mustard
- Measure ingredients into a small bowel, mix and emulsify. Pour over the salad just prior to serving.

Ingredient	Calories	Total fat	Sat Fat	Carbs	Protein	Sodium	Fiber
Olive oil	178.5	20.25	2.7	0	0	0	0
Vinegar	2.5	0	0	1	0	0	0
Mustard	2.5	0	0	0	0	70	0
Totals[8]	183.5	20.25	2.7	1	0	70	0

---

[8] All recipe totals are per serving.

I recommend unsalted, unprocessed peanut butter. Health food stores often have fresh ground peanut butter available. There is a big difference between fresh ground peanut butter and processed. For those who can't eat nuts I would suggest something like a soy burger (e.g. Boca burger) or chicken patty with no bread, or a regular hamburger, along with some fruit. When a peanut butter and jelly is recommended, you could substitute a turkey on whole wheat sandwich (can add mustard and/or a little mayonnaise).

Ingredient	Calories	Total fat	Sat Fat	Carbs	Protein	Sodium	Fiber
Peanut butter (per tblspn)	94	8	2	3	4	3	5
Jelly (tblspn)	56	0	0	13.8	0.1	6	0.2
Whole wheat bread (2 slices)	138	1.9	0.4	23.1	7.25	264	3.8
Totals	288	9.9	2.4	39.9	11.35	273	9

Remember, fruit juice or canned fruit is not the same thing as the real thing—never substitute apple juice for an apple.

Tuna noodle is an easy, no-bake preparation that really hits the spot after the first two days of **The Method**. You could substitute other pasta dishes like spaghetti with a plain sauce (less fat), but the tuna adds some welcome protein. I guess you could make meatballs but the fat would be higher and the dish would be harder to prepare. The recipe for the **tuna noodle** is as follows (will serve two):

- 1 can albacore tuna in water
- ¾ pound macaroni (I prefer spaghetti, but you could use any other pasta)

- 3 tablespoons mayonnaise[9]
- 3 tablespoons sweet relish
- Optional: 1 teaspoon Dijon mustard, hot pepper flakes, and/or pickled hot pepper.
- Cook the pasta. Mix the condiments with the tuna, add to the pasta.
- Dig in!

Ingredient	Calories	Total fat	Sat Fat	Carbs	Protein	Sodium	Fiber
Tuna	166	7.2	1.1	0	23.6	352	3
Macaroni	634	2.7	0.4	127.8	21.9	12	4.1
Mayonnaise	155	17.5	2.4	0	0	109.5	0
Relish	29	0.1	0	7.9	0	182	0.2
Totals	984	27.5	3.9	135.7	45.5	655.5	4.3

The **baked potato** is another simple main course. As the potato bakes, steam the broccoli (could also use spinach). When cooked, split the potato, add 1 tablespoon of butter and mix it well into the hot flesh. Add 1 ounce of cheddar cheese. Place the spinach over the top. Enjoy.

Ingredient	Calories	Total fat	Sat Fat	Carbs	Protein	Sodium	Fiber
Potato	278	0.4	0.1	63.2	7.5	30	6.6
Broccoli	30	0	0	6	2	29	2
Butter	102	12	7.3	0	0	82	0
Cheese	114	9	6	0	7	176	0
Totals	524	21.4	13.4	69.2	16.5	317	8.6

I never could eat cottage cheese and a canned peach-half on a soggy piece of iceberg lettuce—that used to be a favorite appetizer in cheap restaurants or cafeterias when I was a kid. However, cottage cheese and peaches has become one of my staple breakfasts. I don't worry about the fat in the cottage cheese, but if you do, use low fat cottage cheese, or if you're especially fanatical, wash the cheese

---

[9] You could use artificial or low fat but then you'd be violating one of the commandments: <u>Eat real food.</u>

curds draining them of the excess fat. This is the only time that I eat canned fruit. I prefer the peaches in heavy syrup, but you can cut calories by using light peaches.

Ingredient	Calories	Total fat	Sat Fat	Carbs	Protein	Sodium	Fiber
Cottage cheese	216	9	6	5	26	850	0
Peaches	136	0	0	37	1	13	3
Totals	352	9	6	42	27	163	3

You will notice that I have included eggs twice a week. Cholesterol was first implicated in arteriosclerosis in the 1940's and recommendations were made in the early 1970's to decrease the consumption of eggs. While one egg yolk contains 230 grams of cholesterol, it also contains high amounts of lecithin that has the ability to attach to cholesterol and other fats.   In fact, lecithin is sold as a dietary supplement to help the body absorb fat-soluble nutrients and excrete cholesterol.   It's important not to overcook the eggs (as in frying) because the high heat will destroy the lecithin. As mentioned before, the amino acid ratio in eggs makes them the most completely absorbed protein.   You probably could substitute egg-beaters, but once again, you're probably better off with the whole, natural food than the artificial.[10]

Ingredient	Calories	Total fat	Sat Fat	Carbs	Protein	Sodium	Fiber
1 egg	74	5	1.6	0.4	6	70	0

When you eat soup on day six you can buy a can or mix, but remember to read the labels. Better yet, make your own soup.

---

[10] Commandment 5: **Don't try to fake out your body! Eat real food.**

Pea soup (serves 2):

- 1 tablespoon butter
- 1 10 oz bag or box of frozen baby peas (or 4 cups shelled, fresh)
- Sauté peas in butter, add salt and pepper
- Add 1 tablespoon chopped mint
- 2 teaspoons of vegetable bouillon[11] reconstituted with 4 cups of boiling water
- Add water to pea mixture and simmer for 20-30 minutes
- Puree in blender or with immersion blender
- Taste test, add more mint etc.
- Finish with 1 tablespoon of cream or yogurt

Ingredient	Calories	Total fat	Sat Fat	Carbs	Protein	Sodium	Fiber
Butter	51	5.8	3.6	0	0	41	0
Peas	109	0.5	0.1	19.5	7.4	159	6
Mint	1	0	0	0.2	0	1	0.2
Bouillon	10	0	0	1	1	560	2
Cream	26	2.8	1.7	0.2	0.2	3	0
Totals	197	9.1	5.4	20.9	8.6	764	8.2

Curried carrot soup:

- 2 tablespoon extra virgin olive oil
- 1 small leek, white part only, diced (about 1 tablespoon)
- 1 pound peeled, diced carrots
- Sauté the vegetables in the olive oil till soft and lightly browned
- Add 1 teaspoon curry powder and salt and pepper

---

[11] "Better than Bouillon" from www.superiortouch.com. You could substitute fresh stock or chicken stock, or other bouillon cubes.

- Add 4 cups reconstituted vegetable stock (as above)
- Simmer for 20-30 minutes
- While simmering vegetables prepare 1/2 cup couscous (add couscous to 2/3 cup boiling water, turn off heat, cover pan with tight lid and allow to sit for 5 minutes, then fluff with a fork)
- Puree the carrot soup, adjust seasonings
- Add couscous to pureed soup
- Finish with 2 tablespoon plain yogurt, stir to combine
- Heat and serve

Ingredient	Calories	Total fat	Sat Fat	Carbs	Protein	Sodium	Fiber
Olive oil	119	13.5	1.8	0	0	0	0
Leek	14	0.1	0	3.1	0.3	4	0.4
Carrots	93	0.5	0.1	21.7	2.1	156	6.4
Bouillon	10	0	0	1	1	560	2
Couscous	163	0.3	0.1	33.5	5.5	4	2.2
Curry powder	6	0.3	0	1.2	0.2	1	0.7
Yogurt	9	0.2	0.1	1	0.7	10	0
Totals	414	14.9	2.1	61.5	9.8	735	10.2

Spinach macaroni:

- 1 cup acini di pepe, or other small macaroni, cooked in 1 quart salted water.
- In sauté pan melt 1 tablespoon butter in 1 tablespoon olive oil.
- Add 1 clove crushed garlic and hot pepper flakes.
- Slowly simmer, do not burn. Draws out the sweetness of the garlic and melds with the heat of the pepper.
- Add 1 package (10 ounces) washed baby spinach, allow to wilt.
- Add 1 teaspoon vegetable bouillon melted in ½ cup of water.
- Drain macaroni and add to cooked spinach.

- Grate ½ cup (2 ounces) parmesan cheese over mixture and serve.

Ingredient	Calories	Total fat	Sat Fat	Carbs	Protein	Sodium	Fiber
Macaroni	195	0.8	0.1	39.2	6.7	4	1.3
Butter	51	5.8	3.6	0	0	41	0
Olive oil	60	6.7	0.9	0	0	0	0
Garlic	2	0	0	0.5	0.1	0	0
Spinach	65	1.1	0.2	10.3	8.1	224	6.2
Bouillon	5	0	0	0.5	0.5	280	1
Parmesan	111	7	5	1	10	454	0
Totals	489	21.4	9.8	80.4	25.4	1003	3.6

Be Flexible

Any diet that you try to follow should have flexibility. **The Method** is no exception. When you become familiar with the reasoning behind the recommendations, you can make your own substitutions wisely. For example, you should not eat two protein meals back to back, or eat carbohydrate meals in successive nights. It would seem to be common sense that if you are being fairly restrictive, you should spread out the rewards to minimize your cravings.

To summarize **The Method**:

- Keep the 10 commandments.
- Find an accurate method to count calories.[12]
- Don't let any meal exceed 500 calories.
- Substitute liberally, but restrict the fats.
- Don't eat dessert, except maybe a few cookies once a week.
- Realize that it will be impossible to expect the same results if you eat out. However, if you must, be aware and beware!

---

[12] www.youfooddigest.com

12

Further Thoughts

By now, if <u>Set Point</u> has been successful, you will have a greater understanding of what influences your diet and ultimately your weight. Lifestyles, societal and personal attitudes, along with the foods you eat, are all factors that must be addressed for proper weight management. Ultimately only you can control what you put in your mouth. Your mother, father, husband, school, boss, genetics, friends or television didn't force you to eat that extra piece of coconut cream pie. Perhaps that's being too blunt or obvious, but cutting through all the fancy diet books and pop-psychology: <u>if you eat more than you burn up you will gain weight, and remarkably, if you burn up more than you eat, you will lose weight.</u> It really couldn't be stated much simpler.

Before you throw the book down however, look around, you aren't alone in your struggles. For this reason it is important to seek out like-minded individuals, not only joining together in diet support groups, but also to understand and hopefully emulate the habits of those who maintain their weight in a healthy manner. I almost said to emulate those whom you would like to look like, however caffeine, cigarettes, cocaine and other stimulants including diet drugs, and plastic surgery seem to be the staples of models and actors. Don't be fooled! We all get a little thicker around the middle as we age. Because of this fact, I would suggest that it is unnatural not to. It is important to recognize that a healthy weight beneficially influences overall health and well-being.

Understand that a healthy weight doesn't mean being thin. Great athletes tend to be thick because it is necessary to have trunk strength to support powerful legs and shoulders. Traditional eastern philosophies have always painted and sculpted their adepts with a larger middle, to convey the notion of being grounded. It is only modern man that elevates the narrow waisted, and puffed out chested or breasted person. It is not so hard to imagine what would happen to a doll whose weight is mainly in the upper regions—chest and head. It would be unstable, unable to stand and/or easily knocked over. What does that say about societies whose people minimize the natural, solid, earth-bound portions of themselves and worship the higher ego and thinking functions?

Body Types

I don't want to alarm anyone, but we're not all built the same. Therefore, it would be unreasonable to assume that we would all look the same or experience the same difficulties in maintaining weight. This is not a modern concept, though today we classify three main body types: the **ectomorph** (thin and wiry), the **mesomorph** (muscular) and the **endomorph** (fat or fleshy). Each type responds to food and exercise differently. No amount of weight training and diet will make an ectomorph as muscular as the mesomorph who complains: "I don't like to exercise because it makes me too big." The endomorph, on the other hand just has to look at food in order to "pack on the pounds." These body types are not mutually exclusive as there are an infinite number of combinations of them. We actually have always understood this fact.

Hippocrates believed that man's temperament was controlled by specific body fluids or humours: phlegm (phlegma), yellow bile (cholos), blood (sanguis), and black bile (melas cholos). Health depended upon the proper balance of the humours. Dis-ease was considered the result of an imbalance—with a predominance of one humour over the others. While humoral theory most often considered personality, each humour also determined a particular body type. The **phlegmatic** corresponds to the endomorphic type who is prone to water retention, poor circulation, hypothyroidism and slow metabolism. Although he may work slowly, he is deliberate and will persevere. While diet remains important, the phlegmatic should also commit himself to increasing his activity—walking more.

The **choleric** person is usually an ectomorph. One who has a choleric temperament tends to be nervous and sensitive and is easily offended. She is interested in presenting herself in the best light and therefore she is strong willed, sharp minded and concerned with appearance. These traits tend to keep the choleric thin and even prone to anorexia nervosa. The **sanguine** temperament makes one active, impulsive and superficially passionate. He directs much of his attention to what is outside of himself—his environment and his appearance. He is muscular because of his active nature and he would be considered a mesomorph. Finally, the **melancholic** person is introspective and passionate but is slow to motivate and prone to depression. Usually the temperaments are combined to explain the multiple variations of personality types (e.g. melancholic-phlegmatic).

Intensity of feelings (sensitivity) and drive (motivation)			
High	Low		
Choleric	Melancholic	Strong	Emotional Stability
Sanguine	Phlegmatic	Weak	

In India, Ayurveda has been practiced for 5000 years.[1] Vedic science delineates three primary life forces or humours: **vata** (air, wind), **pitta** (fire, bile) and **kapha** (water, phlegm). Personality, temperament and appearance are the result of the unique interplay of the 3 forces in each individual. Usually however, one humour is predominant: vata (dry, light, agitated—ectomorph), pitta (sharp, hot, passionate—mesomorph) and kapha (cold, moist, heavy—endomorph).

In the past, traditional medical sciences tried to explain why people were different and therefore why they should be treated individually. For weight management it is important to note that we all have predispositions which must be recognized, enabling us to best manipulate our own diets.[2] Know thyself. For example, the endomorph-phlegmatic-kapha should avoid most mucous producing dairy products, water retaining salty foods, heavy (red) meats and white flour and rice products. Sounds familiar, doesn't it? The overweight mesomorph-sanguine-pitta needs to control his

---

[1] The "science of life" as detailed in <u>Ayurvedic Healing</u>, Dr. David Frawley O.M.D. Passage Press, Salt Lake City, Utah, 1989.

[2] Recall that both US and Canadian nutritional recommendations have been updated to get away from the one-size-fits-all mentality of the past.

appetite by avoiding sugar, high protein foods, as well as oils. The diet should include lots of fresh fruits and vegetables. The ectomorph-choleric-vata type often eats because of stress and worry. One should avoid stimulants like caffeine, dyes and artificial flavorings, and refined sugars and carbohydrates.

Using the knowledge of body types can be very helpful when choosing foods, spices and supplements. The information I have just given is by no means definitive. I am trying to make you aware of some concepts that can be researched if you are interested. What follows are some general observations and dietary enhancements that you can try. Consulting a health care practitioner, naturopath, herbalist, nutritionist or Ayurvedic practitioner may also be beneficial. In the end however, it's your choice.

Spice It Up

Most people realize that adding spices to food makes it more palatable. Someone is considered a "good cook" because she uses quality ingredients, prepares the food with a deft hand and adds the proper proportion of spices. One of the reasons that meat is so prevalent in the modern, Western diet is because it needs little spice. Therefore it is easy and quick to prepare, and as long as the quality is comparable, meat tends to be very consistent (something you can count on).[3]

Even though most of us prefer them cooked, eating vegetables when they are fresh and raw is the best way to get the nutrients they contain. I remember turning my nose up at the canned peas that my mother served. While frozen

---

[3] That is why most fast-food restaurants are burger and chicken joints.

spinach was barely acceptable, pale, soggy broccoli was a kid's worst nightmare. As I got older I noticed that cultures that ate little meat were proficient at preparing vegetables. When we first looked at Indian or Middle Eastern cookbooks my wife and I were intimidated by the variety of spices that were used. Yet once we acquired and became familiar with a few of the basic spices, which are now readily available, the preparation of curries and other spicy concoctions became simple. By the way, Americans do crave spices and as proof, we eat more mustard than any other spice except black pepper.

In more traditional cultures, food and medicine are two sides of the same coin.[4]   Herbs and spices are used for their medicinal properties as well as for food preservation. Spices fall into two broad categories. **Heating** spices stimulate digestion and include black pepper, cinnamon, hot/red pepper, ginger, mustard, cumin, fenugreek, and cloves. They are used to increase digestive fire and thereby relieve gas, and constipation. **Cooling** spices are excellent body cleansers as well as being good for digestion.   Cooling spices include turmeric, coriander, fennel, nutmeg and cardamom. As a spice, coriander comes as seeds or ground into a powder. In its fresh leaf form it is called cilantro.

Most of the time various spices are combined when added to vegetable and rice dishes. Curry powder is composed of ground coriander, red chili, cumin, mustard, fenugreek, black

---

[4] Modern research is proving the same thing. Cumin seems to have antimicrobial and anti-diabetic effects. Cinnamon increases insulin activity and has antioxidant properties. Ginger increases gastric motility and decreases nausea in post-surgical and seasick patients. It also has anti-inflammatory activity and decreases platelet aggregation (the cause of most heart attacks). Cayenne pepper is an antioxidant and increases metabolism. Turmeric decreases the bad cholesterol (LDL) as well as skin and stomach tumors.

pepper and turmeric. Adding spices to your diet recipes makes them more interesting and satisfying. Don't be afraid to experiment, because then, in a real sense, the whole world of food will open up for you.

Nuts and Seeds

Nuts and seeds can be eaten as tasty and simple snacks, and can be added to many different recipes. Because nuts are high in fat, they have been considered a no-no in most reducing diets. More recently however, evidence has shown they have remarkable health benefits. Research published over ten years ago found that individuals who ate nuts more than five times per week had only 52% of the risk for a heart attack than those who ate nuts less than once a week.[5] This study has been revisited in the last five years and has continued to show a highly significant protective effect of nuts on both the risk of heart attack and death from cardiovascular disease.[6]

The reason for this effect is that nuts are high in mono- and poly-unsaturated fat and plant sterols. The Mediterranean diet has been shown to be healthy because olive oil is also high in mono-unsaturated fat.[7] The nuts most often studied have been almonds, walnuts and pecans. Unfortunately we usually think of nuts as being canned, oil roasted, salted and sugar coated—in other words—processed. The nuts that are being studied and recommended are raw and/or dry

---

[5] Adventist Health Study published in the *Archives of Internal Medicine*, July 1992.

[6] The Iowa Women's Study has also demonstrated the same protective effect of nuts.

[7] Mono-unsaturated fatty acids have been shown to lower bad cholesterol (LDL) and raise good cholesterol (HDL).

roasted without added preservatives. Therefore it is best to buy nuts in a health food store or co-op, or in the shell. Obviously I am not suggesting that you sit in front of the TV and mindlessly polish off a can of salted, mixed nuts. Add nuts to your diet, but in reasonable quantities.

Seeds are another source of protective plant sterols and they are also high in protein, fiber and minerals like zinc, potassium and iron. Pumpkin, sesame and sunflower seeds are the ones most often ingested. Sunflower seeds are especially good as a protein supplement, but they should be eaten in small amounts due to their calorie content. Flax and psyllium seeds are a rich source of essential fatty acids and they alleviate constipation.

Supplementation

The proper use of food products, either as whole food or as supplements, can be beneficial for your health.   Food should be your medicine.   The sterols in nuts are more commonly called phytosterols, which are found in all plants. Soy and soy products are rich in phytosterols which helps to explain their healthful effects. When taken as a supplement phytosterols, along with a slightly modified, weight loss diet, can lower cholesterol 25-40%. This number is comparable to that obtained with daily use of statin drugs.[8]   As has already been mentioned, fiber, which is plentiful in fresh fruits and vegetables, is an important protector against colon cancer and will help to absorb and excrete dietary fat and cholesterol.

----

[8] See an excellent review of this subject in The New 8-Week Cholesterol Cure, by Robert Kowalski, Harper Collins Publishers, New York, New York, 2002.

Hopefully you have learned that we eat too much processed food, and that obesity makes us susceptible to many diseases. However, most of us ignore the fact that we are fed devitalized foods grown in nutrient poor soils that have to be enriched with fertilizers. To protect the crops grown in these artificially enhanced conditions, <u>4.5 billion pounds of pesticides are used yearly</u> in the United States. In the early years, our country was covered in 18 to 25 inches of topsoil. This number has been reduced to less than 6 inches in most of the "bread-basket" of the mid-West. Is there any wonder where the dust storms of the thirties found their scorched earth?

In an elegant presentation, Ronald Wright discussed the downfall of numerous powerful civilizations. While disease and outside conquest were sometimes implicated, too often the cultures misused and contaminated their environments through poor farming and resource management. "Farming achieved quantity at the expense of quality: more food and more people, but seldom better nourishment or better lives. People gave up a broad array of wild foods for a handful of starchy roots and grasses—wheat, barley, rice, potatoes and maize (corn). As we domesticated plants, the plants domesticated us. In the matter of our food, we have grown as specialized, and therefore as vulnerable, as a saber-toothed cat."[9] The great city-states spilled over into their surroundings and their soils were ruined by over-irrigation and crop redundancy.

Therefore besides the faulty eating habits described throughout this book, we have grown used to vitamin-poor foods that need to be enriched. So obvious is the need for supplementation to fill in our nutritional gaps that we spend

---

[9] A Short History of Progress, by Ronald Wright, p. 47. House of Anansi Press, Inc. Toronto, Ontario, Canada, 2004.

$9 billion a year on these products. Beware and be aware. Not all vitamins are the same. I remember when nutritionist Robert Jensen D. Ch. burned certain vitamin pills on a plate. What remained was coal-tar, a petroleum based substance. Choose your supplements wisely yet judiciously. Eat real food—buy organic and local as much as possible.[10] Let food be your medicine. Follow the 10 Commandments.

Fasting

Fasting can be most broadly defined as eating foods that are at least one step lighter in substance than what is normally consumed: avoiding meat if you are a meat eater, eating raw fruits and vegetables if you are a vegetarian, going on a juice fast if your diet is already light enough, and finally the traditional water fast. Fasting has been recommended as a healing therapy for thousands of years by the classical physicians Hippocrates, Galen and Paracelsus. Perhaps they observed that animals do not eat when sick. As Paavo Airola explained:

> During a prolonged fast (after the first three days), your body will live on its own substance. When it is deprived of needed nutrition, particularly of proteins and fats, it will burn and digest its own tissues by the process of *autolysis*, or self-digestion. But your body will not do it indiscriminately! In its wisdom—and here lies the secret of the extraordinary effectiveness of fasting as curative and rejuvenative therapy!—your body will *first* decompose and burn those cells and tissues which are diseased, damaged, aged or dead.[11]

---

[10] Information at www.organicconsumers.com.

Not only has fasting been used in the healing arts for thousands of years, it has been recognized to be an important technique for spiritual awakening for an even longer period.[12]   All the great religious traditions mention fasting in their rituals and scripture whether it be the ascetic practices of the Buddha prior to his awakening, Christ's forty days of fasting in the desert prior to His Transfiguration, or the forty day fast of Moses before his descent from Mount Sinai carrying the tablets of stone. Fasting for the month of Ramadan is one of Islam's five pillars of faith, demonstrating disregard for earthly goods and the belief that Allah will provide. There must be some spiritual value in "lightening your load" both physically and mentally.

There are numerous ways to fast and as mentioned above, the easiest way is to eat a progressively lighter diet in a step-wise fashion. It wouldn't be wise to go from the "supersize me" North American diet to a water fast. Before you consider a fast it is especially important to seek advice from your health care professional. Unfortunately most medical doctors are not skilled in this area, and you may have to seek out a naturopath or holistic nutritionist. I bring up this thought because a cleansing fast may be an excellent way to jumpstart your new way of eating—once again **changing your set point**.

---

[11] How to Get Well, Paavo Airola N.D., Ph.D., p. 215. Health Plus Publishers, Sherwood, Oregon, 1974.

[12] Of course priests were the early healers, and temples were originally healing sanctuaries, so this relationship should come as no surprise.

Beware of terrified protein

As this chapter may sound a little radical I might as well complete the thought. Protein is memory. When we eat protein we are eating the memory of another living organism. Do you really think it's wise to eat factory-farmed poultry that are raised in cramped cages being pecked by other frightened, frustrated birds? What about feed-lot cattle who live in filth? If we can smell death that permeates from the slaughter houses (remember they're located far from human habitation for a reason) don't you think the animals can smell it?

"But animals don't think and feel." Say that to a pet-owner sitting next to, and trying to reassure, her trembling dog in the vet's waiting room. The hormones and waste products (lactic acid and ammonia) secreted into the frightened animals' systems and getting incorporated into their protein may not be the best stuff to consume. Understand I'm not saying one needs to be a vegetarian, but you should consider the source of your meat. When it is presented in bright, plastic-wrapped, sterile packages alongside hundreds of similar appearing pieces under a sign from which a jovial bull or smiling tuna beckons—beware. Maybe those smiles are trying to hide the terror.

Don't be fooled

Try to answer the question: what is important to you? Why do you want to lose weight? Hopefully the answer is to feel better and to feel better about yourself. However, too often we view ourselves in the funhouse mirror of the media. Do not forget that the media and marketing are some of the leading causes of the obesity epidemic. Isn't it ironic that on the one hand we are sucked in by slick ad campaigns for every kind of empty calorie and chain restaurant, yet at the same time we are fed a steady diet of abnormally thin, surgically altered media stars who make us feel inadequate because we don't look like them? I remember one of the famous ultra-thin supermodels extolling the virtues of cigarettes, coffee and cocaine. It comes with a price!

An incredible amount of money is spent to make unhealthy foods attractive to you. Throughout this book I have mentioned governmental bias that keeps the food industry humming. The diet industry is no slouch either. Wall Street is constantly on the prowl for the next great diet plan or book. In a New York Times article, the marketing of a new diet book from "Jorge Cruise, a suntanned fitness guru from San Diego" was detailed. The vice-president of merchandising for Barnes and Noble Bob Wietrak asserted, "This will probably be the No. 1 diet book for 2005, without a doubt."[13] We are always being marketed to, but never forget **all diets work. All diets are meant to fail**. Don't be fooled by the pretty face or the wash-board abs—you've got to do the work. **To change your set point you must change your mindset!**

Every corporation and especially those in the pharmaceutical industry are determined to cash in. "Everybody is just foaming at the mouth to make money from obesity drugs."[14] Medicare has said that it will now pay for effective obesity treatments and drug industry experts believe that a weight-loss pill could have annual sales far surpassing the $12 billion generated by the cholesterol treating statin drug Lipitor. Companies make you fat so that they can sell you

---

[13] New York Times, Sunday April 17, 2005.

[14] Dr. Donna Ryan, an obesity researcher affiliated with Louisiana State University, which has received millions of dollars in government and industry grants. Quoted in the New York Times, April 5, 2005.

the drugs to make you thin. Stop the madness! Eat fresh, nutritious, healthy foods at a calorie level that is less than you burn up daily.

Stress Again

One cannot underestimate the effects of stress on health. Researchers have concluded that when all other factors are considered (e.g. diet, economic status and access to care), the reason that Americans consume more health care dollars and die younger than other first world nations is the stress level of the society. These stresses include how hard we work, the noise level we live with, the constant exposure to electro-magnetic radiation and the need to "succeed". The next time you are playing with your kids, concentrating on an interesting project, hiking in the woods or lying on the beach ask yourself why you aren't thinking about food. Whether you're distracted or just enjoying yourself, the bottom line is you aren't as stressed-out. When you are more satisfied, more content and more joy-filled, the stresses of life will melt away—and maybe, just maybe—the pounds will too!

Where You Are

Finally, I need to return to some of the basic principles of the book, and ultimately of life:

- Know thyself. Heal thyself.
- Be honest with yourself. Beware and be aware.
- This is a lifetime project.
- Be patient with yourself and relax.
- Lighten up.

In the end it is important to understand that **you are precisely where you are supposed to be in order to learn what you are meant to learn**. Adapt, adjust and acclimatize, for all life is change. Every journey begins with the first step. Where do you want to go?

Invitation

Sit on the throne of God. It's still warm.
You have a place at the Table.
There's plenty to eat

Why are you still hungry?

ISBN 142510179-8